CIRCUMCISION IS A FRAUD:

AND THE COMING LEGAL RECKONING

BY PETER W. ADLER, MA, JD

DEDICATION

With love to my mother, Dorothy, who encouraged me to write, and to my wonderful family: my wife Gail, who has been so endlessly helpful and supportive over the seven years it took me to develop the ideas in this book; our children Carolyn, Geoffrey, and Christy; and our adorable grandchildren Annabelle, Will, and Nate.

FOREWORD

Are you aware that America is the only nation in which it is thought necessary to operate for non-religious reasons on newborn baby boys to remove the foreskin, a normal functional body part with which every boy is born? Why do Americans accept and approve of this practice? Have you ever wondered how this came to be? Does America have some secret information which is denied to other developed nations? How are boys affected by this surgical amputation? Is it beneficial or is it harmful? How do doctors view the practice? Why did it come into existence? How is it sustained? Should anything be done to change it?

Peter Adler, J.D., a legal scholar and a professor of international law, whom I have known for many years, had his first personal experience with circumcision when his son was born. His experience opened his eyes and aroused his curiosity. He is probably the most intelligent and best educated man I know. He now has thoroughly investigated the practice of infant circumcision in America in several influential scholarly law review articles in which various medical and legal issues regarding the circumcision of boys have been reviewed.[1,2,3]

The subject matter embraces both medical issues and legal matters presented for lay persons. He may have been aided with medical matters, since his wife, Gail, is a professor of medicine. Professor Adler has now written an easy-to-read narrative, detailing his findings for the general public, in which he answers the questions presented above and much more.

He provides the history of the practice, examines the medical effects, and contrasts the views of Europeans and Americans. Professor Adler shows that circumcision of boys has no medical indication, is non-therapeutic, non-prophylactic, and medically unnecessary. He documents the

---

1   Adler PW. Is It Lawful to Use Medicaid to Pay for Circumcision? *J Law & Med.* 2011-12;19(2): 335-53. <researchgate.net/publication/221818830>.

2   Adler PW. Is Circumcision Legal? *Rich J L & Pub Int.* 2013;16(3):439-86. <scholarship.richmond.edu/cgi/viewcontent.cgi?article=1265&context=jolpi>.

3   Adler PW, Van Howe RS, Wisdom T, Daase F. Is Circumcision a Fraud? *Cornell J L & Public Policy.* 2020-11;30(1):45-107. <lawschool.cornell.edu/research/JLPP/upload/Adler-et-al-final.pdf>.

certain pain, harm, injury, and loss of numerous protective, immunological, sexual, and sensory functions caused by amputation of the most
sensitive part of the penis.

He shows that many American physicians and their medical trade associations omit information about the nature and function of the foreskin
and do not tell the parents of newborn boys and the American public the
truth about the practice of circumcision, so as to preserve the large income stream they derive from it. He also suggests possible remedies.

Professor Adler's book should be essential reading for prospective
parents, grandparents, and caregivers, medical doctors (especially family
doctors, pediatricians, obstetricians, and urologists), lawyers who are
considering taking legal action related to the circumcision of boys, and
judges.

George Hill, Vice-President
Doctors Opposing Circumcision
January 14, 2022

TABLE OF CONTENTS

Prologue

On April 7, 1987, after laboring on medications, my wife gave birth to our son Geoffrey, and the physician who delivered him pronounced him healthy. We expected to take him home from the hospital shortly thereafter, as we had previously taken our daughter home soon after she was born, but later the next day a physician confronted us with an unexpected question.

"The Question"

My wife (a physician and researcher at Harvard Medical School's Brigham & Women's Hospital, and now a professor of medicine there) was nursing our newborn boy, and I was just happy to be with them – content, proud, and daydreaming. My thoughts were interrupted by the loud voice of a physician coming from behind the door he was opening: "Have you decided yet whether to have your son circumcised or not?" The question took me completely by surprise. My wife and I had never discussed circumcision. I thought to myself that it seems like a bad idea to cut off part of a penis. On the other hand, the doctor's question suggested that it was a good idea, that there must be some medical basis for circumcising a boy, and that my wife and I should have considered it beforehand. In any event, he was telling us to consider it and to decide now.

The physician suddenly appeared standing close to me in the middle of the room. He faced me, with his back turned to my wife, who was nursing our son on a bed to my left. He was a middle-aged man, a physician we had not met before. He was wearing a long white lab coat with the name of the hospital and a name tag that said DOCTOR. He looked very official and spoke authoritatively as physicians are wont to do.

I said, "My wife and I have never thought about it." I then thought to myself, my wife is a physician, and she is very practical, whereas I was a philosophy major and graduate student, I am not so practical, and I know nothing about medicine. I turned to my wife and said, "This sounds important: you are a physician, you should join the conversation." Meaning: this is a joint decision and please help me make it! Ever since that day, my wife has been the extended family's Chief Medical Officer, making recommendations when anyone in the family has any medical problem. She replied with what I only later realized was a vacant look: "You have a penis, sweetheart, you decide." The doctor made no effort to include my wife – he never once looked at her or at my son while talking to me – even though she was a physician at the same hospital, she had given birth to our son the day before, we were both our son's parents, and he was the boy that the physician was offering to circumcise. She went back to blissfully nursing him. I later learned that soliciting parental permission for circumcision is called "The Question."

"THE TALK"

The doctor then asked whether I was familiar with circumcision. I knew nothing about it, but I had heard it called a "snip." I visualized a single snip of a small and useless part of the foreskin of my son's penis, with scissors that somehow were not sharp. I said, "No." Harvard hospitals and physicians are among the best in the world, my wife and brother, an emergency room doctor, being cases in point. I thought to myself, this man must know more about circumcision than anyone alive. I should hear him out, hear what medical reason there is for cutting off part of the penis. I focused intently on what he told me, and it made an indelible impression on me.

The doctor said that circumcision is a simple procedure, and that in the United States about 55% of parents elect it for their sons. Sometimes I am a contrarian, but I thought that since the majority of parents in the U.S. opt for circumcision, perhaps I should as well.

He continued that the American Academy of Pediatrics (AAP), a medical organization for pediatricians – which I had never heard of but had no reason to doubt knew what it was talking about – has reviewed the medical literature and does not recommend circumcision. That seemed a reason to say "no." I later learned that the AAP issues circumcision guidelines for physicians and the American public, which it has revised from time to time. If nurses and/or physicians tell parents anything about circumcision, which they do less than half the time, they usually give the parents a summary of the AAP guidelines then in effect ("The Talk").

The doctor then said that the foreskin of the penis covers the glans or head of the penis and protects it for life. Circumcision removes all or most of the foreskin and exposes the glans. The mix of urine and feces in diapers can cause an infection, resulting in a narrowing of the opening at the end of the penis. I only later learned that this happens often, 17.9% of the time. That seemed to be another reason to say "no."

He continued that the procedure has potential medical benefits, which he explained means that it reduces the risk of males contracting certain diseases. According to the American Academy of Pediatrics, medical studies show that circumcised boys have 1% fewer urinary tract infections (UTIs) during the first year of life than boys who have a foreskin. That is not a justification for circumcision, however, he said, because urinary tract infections are relatively rare, and they can be treated with antibiotics. (I later learned that girls get UTIs more frequently than boys do during early childhood, and of course no one suggests that as a reason to cut girls' genitals.) That seemed yet another reason to say "no."

The physician said that according to the American Academy of Pediatrics, circumcision slightly reduces the risk of penile cancer. I visualized a penis riddled by cancer. Penile cancer sounded like a terrible disease to be avoided at all costs. He provided a statistic that I do not recall, but it showed that the risk of penile cancer is extremely low. The physician said that circumcision is not justified as a preventative measure against penile cancer because it is a rare disease that occurs primarily in old age, and it can be avoided by washing the penis and by not smoking. That seemed to be another reason to say "no."

He then said that according to the American Academy of Pediatrics, circumcision slightly reduces the risk of sexually active adolescent boys and men contracting some sexually transmitted infections. But he said that this is not a justification for circumcision because behavioral factors are more important in causing sexually transmitted infections than having a foreskin, and those diseases can be avoided by being monogamous or by practicing safe sex. That seemed like yet another reason to say "no."

The physician continued. He said that it is customary for parents in the United States to make medical decisions on behalf of their children because they are below the age of consent. Parents should decide whether their son will be circumcised or not. He also said that when making the circumcision decision "in the multicultural society that is the United States" (the phrasing struck me as odd), it is legitimate for parents to take into consideration their own religious, cultural, and personal beliefs in addition to medical reasons.

I asked, "What do you mean by religious reasons?" He said that among some religious groups, it is a religious rite or a tradition to circumcise boys. I said, "I am not religious."

I asked, "What do you mean by cultural reasons?" He said that in some cultures, it is a tradition for boys to be circumcised. That seemed to be a bad reason to circumcise a boy. I said, "I don't care what people in some cultures do." Being of British origin, I am usually not so blunt, but I was starting to get irritated.

I asked, "What do you mean by personal reasons?" He said that sometimes parents elect to have their son circumcised because they prefer the appearance of the circumcised penis. I asked what he meant. He said that when the father is circumcised, often the parents want the son's penis to look like the father's penis. Indeed, I later learned, that is the main reason that parents in the U.S. elect to have their son circumcised.

The physician's statement caught my attention, and it ultimately gave rise to this book. I thought back to torts class during the first semester of law school. Physicians are required to obtain the patient's fully informed consent to perform any medical procedure. Otherwise, the procedure is unlawful, even if the patient needs it. My son is below the age of consent. The physician needs my permission, acting as my son's proxy or legal representative, to circumcise my son. Otherwise, he is not allowed to do the procedure.

Then it suddenly occurred to me that the claim that he had just made – that parents have the right to elect to have part of their son's penis cut away because they prefer the appearance of the circumcised penis – could not be true. I thought to myself that laws are usually of broad application. If a judge ruled that a father had that right, it would follow that a father would also have the right to choose to cut off any other part or parts of his son's body to "match" the father's body. Mothers would have that right too. That could not be possible: there could be no such law.

My thinking was interrupted when the physician asked, "Do you have any questions?" I visualized my son as a young man. I asked, "Can't my son make this decision for himself when he becomes an adult?" The physician replied that the procedure is best performed in infancy. He said that it is more complicated when performed later in life and more costly. He kept talking, but I did not hear what he said because I had tuned him out. He had not answered my question. Obviously, the correct answer was "yes," my son could make the decision for himself when he became an adult. I felt pressured to consent.

MY DECISION

This entire conversation had taken only a few minutes, five at most. Doctors are very busy people, and he was waiting for an answer. He had told me that this medical association, the American Academy of Pediatrics, which he invoked as an authority on circumcision, does not recommend it, and it is not medically justified, but that some parents elect it because of their own religious, cultural, and personal aesthetic preferences. I felt that my job, acting on behalf of my son and as his representative, was to choose whatever would be best for his health, without regard to what I might prefer, if different. And it seemed better that my son should make this decision for himself instead of my making it for him. I reasoned that I could not go wrong by saying "no." I told the doctor emphatically, "No, we do not want our son circumcised."

The conversation had been upsetting, confusing, and threatening. I had felt defensive, for reasons that I could not articulate at the time. In retrospect, I had trusted the physician, but he had told me something untrue. I later realized that this raised the question of whether anything else he was telling me was untrue, and of whether he was disclosing everything that I needed to know about the procedure to make an informed decision about it.

I was comfortable with my decision, and I promptly forgot about this unsettling encounter. We returned home the next day with our whole baby, his body intact, exactly the way he was born, and we and our daughter Carolyn welcomed him into the family.

INCREASING DOUBTS

It took about two decades, or until 2007, for me to question the practice of circumcision again, after I learned that there are charitable organizations opposed to it. In the United States, these include *Doctors Opposing Circumcision, Nurses For the Rights of the Child, Attorneys for the Rights of the Child, Your Whole Baby, Circumcision Resource Center, Catholics Against Circumcision, Jews Against Circumcision,* and *Intact America,* the largest charitable organization in the U.S. working to end unnecessary genital cutting. There are parents in Israel opposed to it as well, even though it is a sacred religious rite among the Jewish people. It would have been helpful had the physician who pitched circumcision to me informed me that the practice is controversial and that there is widespread opposition to it. In fact, *The Bloodstained Men,* a group opposed to circumcision, could have been right outside the hospital where my son had been born protesting the practice, wearing pants with blood stains on them – graphically showing that circumcision is not bloodless or painless as I had assumed – and I would only have learned about it after my son had been circumcised, which is irreversible.

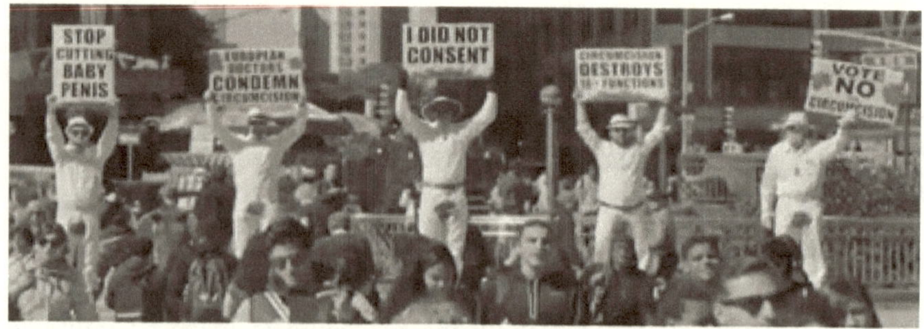

The Bloodstained Men protesting circumcision[4]

---

4   The Bloodstained Men. <bloodstainedmen.com>.

Learning about this opposition reminded me of my discomforting experience in the hospital when the physician had asked me – forced me – to decide whether to have my son circumcised or not. I began to question why people oppose the practice and to learn more about it, as increasing numbers of other people in the U.S. were and are doing. Starting in 2009, I attended several Genital Autonomy symposia where respected professionals from around the world give talks every year promoting genital integrity and opposing unnecessary male, female, and intersex genital cutting. The presentations were eye opening, shocking in fact.

I was surprised to learn that when boys are born in most countries, especially ones that do not have a majority population of Muslims or Jews, physicians leave them genitally intact. Physicians in the United States are thus outliers, even compared to other developed countries, in asking parents whether they want to have their son circumcised or not, and in actually circumcising the majority of boys, most at birth but some later in childhood. Given that circumcision is uncommon in these other countries with advanced healthcare systems, it is not necessary to circumcise any newborn boy, and indeed it is rarely necessary to do so at any time during childhood. Do physicians in the U.S. know something about the desirability of circumcision that physicians in other similar countries do not know? That seemed unlikely. And it seemed odd that physicians worldwide are not in agreement about the subject.

I learned from Marilyn Milos, the mother of the so-called intactivist movement,[5] that circumcision is extremely painful. Up until the 1980s, when my son was born, most doctors did not use any pain control, apparently thinking it would be too much of a hassle for such a "simple" procedure, or mistakenly and counterintuitively believing that babies don't feel pain. Even with drugs to lessen the pain, which often are not used even today (and which unfortunately carry risks of their own), circumcision can still hurt the baby a great deal. Doctors see this and know this, but they do not typically disclose it to parents. The pain also continues after the surgery when the wound is healing.

---

5   Bollinger D. Origins of the Intactivist Movement: A Masculine Foundation. *Men's Sexual Rights.* 2017-11. <researchgate.net/publication/321837170>.

I learned from Robert Van Howe, M.D., the leading U.S. physician-scholar in the field, that cutting off the foreskin of a boy's penis risks more than 50 physical complications. The American Academy of Pediatrics calls most of these complications minor, such as an unsatisfactory cosmetic result, but the owner of the penis might not agree that the complications are minor. Some complications are catastrophic and would destroy any person's life. Dr. Christian Fletcher discussed how he sees an endless line of men wounded by circumcision. It can also be fatal. See Dr. Van Howe's affidavit, Appendix.

I had assumed that the "procedure" – actually, it is a surgical operation – is harmless when it is performed properly. But pain is a harm, loss of the most sensitive part of the penis is a harm, and a scar is evidence of a wound and a harm. Whatever one may think about potential health benefits, then, in terms of their ability to "compensate" for these harms, what should be clear is that circumcision, as a baseline, harms all boys who undergo it and all of the men they become, even when properly performed.

Another presenter discussed how the clamps that physicians use are all dangerous because the physician cannot see exactly what part of a boy's penis is being cut. Psychologists and a psychiatrist discussed how genital cutting can cause psychological problems among adolescents and later in life, when males come to realize what was done to their penis and taken from them, without medical need and without their consent.

The Harvard trained attorney J. Steven Svoboda, Founder and Executive Director of *Attorneys for the Rights of the Child,* an intellectual father of the intactivist movement, suggested scholarly articles for me to read arguing that non-therapeutic (not needed to treat), elective (a choice) circumcision is unethical, according to standard principles used in biomedical ethics, and unlawful, as discussed in this book. It was news to me that the practice even might be unethical and unlawful.

What I learned persuaded me that I had made the right decision for my son. But the parents of newborn boys in the U.S. make the opposite decision and choose to have their son circumcised about 1.5 million times per year. There remains a debate, especially in the United States, about whether boys should be circumcised or not. What is the debate about, and can it be resolved?

Please consider joining this mailing list to learn more about circumcision or genital cutting and about efforts to end it, at

<circumcisionisafraud.com/book>.

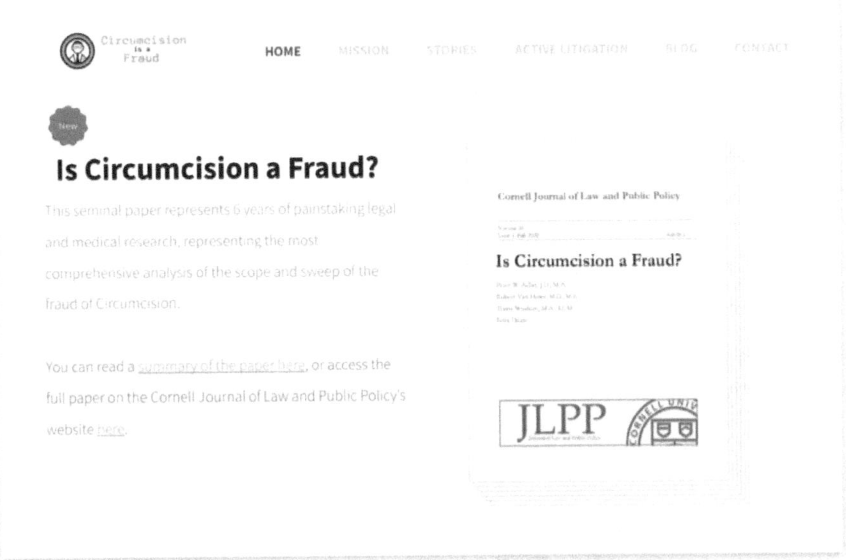

2   "THE DEBATE", THESIS, AND AUDIENCE

"THE DEBATE"

Physicians ordinarily leave living tissue and healthy parts of children's bodies alone. Likewise, physicians in most countries leave boys' and girls' genitals alone and intact, so let us begin there.

As discussed in Part I, the proponents of genital integrity, who are opponents of the unnecessary cutting of a minor's genitals, argue that the human genital prepuce – in males the foreskin of the penis and in females the clitoral hood – is a natural body part that is an essential component of perfect health, and that it is very good for health. Unnecessary genital cutting is bad for health, and it has little prospect of benefiting any boy or man. Regardless, as discussed in Part II, medically unnecessary genital cutting performed without the consent of the person affected by it violates numerous fundamental rules of medical ethics and legal rights of the child. When boys become men, they have the right to decide the fate of the foreskin of their own penis for themselves.

As discussed in Part IV, the proponents of circumcision or genital cutting, who are opponents of genital integrity – primarily physicians in the United States, their hospitals, and their medical associations, as well as religious adherents in some parts of the world – argue the opposite. As they see it, the foreskin is prone to infection and bad for health, and it has no value. Removing the foreskin has many medical benefits, which out-weigh the risks. Regardless, parents have the right to elect to have their son circumcised for any reason, including for religious, cultural, and aes-thetic reasons, and physicians have the right to circumcise boys when the parents do elect it.

	THE FORESKIN	GENITAL CUTTING	WHO DECIDES?	ETHICAL AND LAWFUL?
OPPONENTS	Good for health and valuable	Bad for health	The owner of the penis	No
PROPONENTS	Bad for health and has no value	Good for health	His parents	Yes

Thus, the positions of the proponents of genital integrity or opponents of male genital cutting (as they prefer to call the practice, since they view it as analogous to female and intersex genital cutting) and of the proponents of circumcision (as they prefer to call it) are complete opposites. But the practice must be either good or bad or somewhere in between. And it must be ethical and lawful or not: it cannot be both. How can this extremely longstanding debate be resolved?

This is a controversial topic where emotions run high. Let us defuse the controversy and simplify the analysis by taking parents, physicians, and even boys and the foreskin of the penis out of the equation. Let us hypothesize that a layperson cuts off an adult's healthy finger without his or her consent. That is simply violence – criminal assault and a civil battery (an unlawful touching) – unless the person doing the cutting can justify it, such as by showing that he or she acted in self-defense.

Likewise, as discussed in Chapter 9 (Physicians Bear the Burden of Justifying Genital Cutting), a physician bears the burden of justifying the surgical removal of any part of an adult's body. Except for cosmetic surgery that an adult requests, the physician must determine that the operation is medically necessary and obtain the adult's consent to it. The same rules apply to cutting a minor's genitals. Physicians need to prove that the boy or girl in question needs the operation, and that the operation cannot be deferred until adulthood when the man or woman can consent it.

This book suggests, then, that the arguments opposed to unnecessary genital cutting are correct, whereas the arguments in favor of it by the American medical profession – and the argument by religious adherents that they have the religious right to have it performed – are unpersuasive and indeed indefensible.

Circumcision is not good for the health of boys and men, nor is it completely or almost completely harmless as the U.S. medical profession has long portrayed it. But the case against circumcision does not turn on scientific claims. As the philosopher David Hume wrote, there is a distinction between the descriptive or what "is" and the prescriptive or what "ought" to be. Unnecessary, non-consensual genital cutting is ultimately an ethical and legal matter. Regardless of any debates about health or harmfulness, physicians do not have the right to operate on a healthy boy's genitals any more than they have the right to operate on a health girl's genitals, or to cut off a child's finger, barring a medical emergency. By way of example, even if the medical profession claimed that there were "health benefits" to female genital cutting, no one would accept this as a valid justification for the practice.

Performing an operation on a healthy child crosses a line that physicians are not allowed to cross, no matter what arguments they might advance in favor of it. Therefore, no one should accept any of the great many and, as will be shown, ever-changing possible justifications that the American medical profession has advanced in support of routine male genital cutting, or might in the future.

Genital cutting, when you get right down to it, is a form of violence, regardless of the sex characteristics or gender identity of the affected person. It is violence masquerading as medicine. Physicians and religious adherents have powerful financial and religious incentives to continue the practice and to try to defend it, but they will never be able to do so successfully, as I will endeavor to show. Hence, I suggest that the circumcision debate is over.

A FRAUD?

Thus, physicians have built the circumcision industry by making false claims and by not disclosing the truth about it. The American medical profession falsely portrays it as the simple, painless snip of a useless piece of skin; fails to disclose to parents that it is painful, risky, and inherently harmful; and claims that it has actual or potential medical benefits, when as discussed in this book, it has little prospect of benefiting any boy or man, and any possible benefits can be achieved easily and more safely without the risks and harms of the operation. Therefore, it will never be possible to justify it on medical grounds.

The question then arises, are these physicians in the U.S. and their medical associations making their false claims in good faith, or knowingly? And if the latter, do they intentionally deceive the American public and the parents of newborn boys about it? Is the circumcision industry analogous to the tobacco industry, which used a trade association it supported, The Tobacco Institute, to help the industry portray smoking in a favorable light and to defend it in the face of claims that tobacco is addictive and very bad for health?

That is exactly what the legal scholar Matthew Giannetti argued in a 2000 article. He accused the American Academy of Pediatrics of having issued possibly fraudulent circumcision guidelines in 1989 and 1999 designed to perpetuate the practice and thereby physicians' profits. The reader is likely to be unaware, as I was, that circumcision is a multibillion dollar per year industry, as discussed in Chapter 15 (Undisclosed Conflicts of Interest and Motives to Defraud).

Scholars have shown that the AAP's most recent 2012 guidelines, issued shortly after a German court ruled that circumcision is criminal assault, contain even more extravagant and indefensible claims than the 1999 guidelines that preceded them. The critique of the AAP's 2012 guidelines by thirty-eight physicians and medical ethicists representing pediatric medical associations in Northern Europe, discussed later in this book, is short, easy to read, and devastating.[6]

It occurred to me that the American Academy of Pediatrics could not possibly have believed some of its claims in 2012. I planned to give a talk at the Genital Autonomy conference in Boulder, Colorado in 2015 about how the AAP's 2012 guidelines were intentionally fraudulent or intended to deceive the public and the parents of newborn boys. As I was preparing the talk, though, I thought back to how, when my son was born, my wife was "out of it," and how the physician had ignored her; how he had given me only a few minutes to decide the fate of my son's foreskin, without the benefit of a second opinion; and how he had not disclosed that the foreskin is highly erogenous or any of the risks and harms of the operation. Had he told me any of those things, I would have said "no" even faster and more emphatically than I did. Most parents would say "no" too if told the truth about the practice, such as that it will deprive their son of

6   Frisch M, et al. Cultural Bias in the AAP's 2012 Technical Report and Policy Statement on Male Circumcision. *Pediatrics*. 2013-04-01;131(4):796-800. <pediatrics.aappublications.org/content/131/4/796>.

the most sensitive part of his penis for life; that it risks serious medical complications and can be fatal; that their son might resent having had part of his penis cut off when it was perfectly healthy; and that some parents come to regret having authorized the operation. In short, like the AAP, physicians and nurses, who are medical professionals subject to the rules of medical ethics as well, do not tell the American public or parents the whole truth about the practice.

Over time I started to think about circumcision as a service industry, and about the different parts of running the business, such as how to market this bad thing as a good thing; how to answer difficult questions that the media and parents might have; what to tell parents or to hide from them to persuade them to say "yes"; how to get paid for performing unnecessary surgery; and how to defend the industry from the increasing opposition that it is facing both inside and outside the United States.

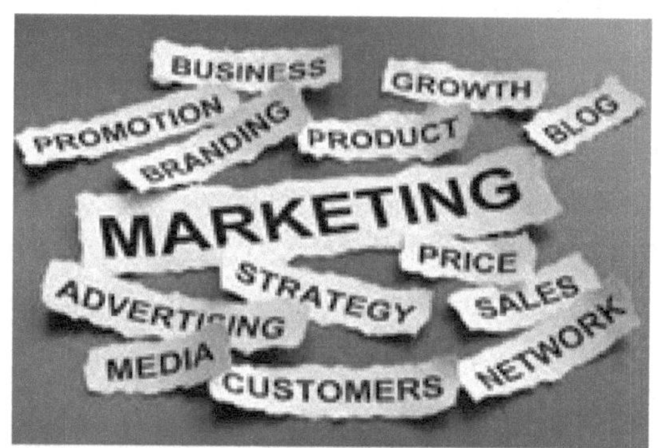

One day boys are born with, and they have, an anatomically correct penis with a foreskin, like most males who have ever lived, and the next day or two it is gone forever. Physicians and their hospitals in turn get paid to take it from them. Thus, physicians take something from boys and men that they typically value, and in any event have the legal right to keep, and in exchange physicians and their hospitals get something that they value, namely money (and as will be shown, lots of it). Physicians in the United States do not circumcise boys because it benefits *the boys and men,* as they claim and as most Americans believe, but because it benefits *themselves and their hospitals.* The more I learned about the practice in the United States, the more I became convinced that it is rotten to the core: it is quack medicine supported by junk science, a scam, a hoax, a fraud.

Part IV considers every argument that I could find that the proponents of circumcision have advanced since 1875 (more than one hundred different claims before 1971 alone) and that they make now in the 21st century. Otherwise, this would not be much of a book. None of them are convincing.

How is circumcision a fraud, expressed as simply as possible? By using various intentional unfair and deceptive practices dating back 150 years, physicians in the United States take the foreskin that males value, want to keep, and have the right to keep, and harm them. Physicians and hospitals thereby enrich themselves at the expense of boys and men whom the physicians have a duty to and swore to protect.

Do boys and men who are angry to have been circumcised and their parents have valid legal claims against the physician and hospital? As shown in this book, yes, they do. And although litigation is an ugly business, litigation considerations are largely favorable to these plaintiffs.

AUDIENCE AND PURPOSE

The book is aimed at three different audiences.

The first is lay people. Hopefully, the book will persuade more parents of newborn boys and older boys to "just say no." Physicians in the U.S. and their medical associations have made clear that they are not going to stop circumcising boys of their own accord, however, so the book also hopes to persuade circumcised boys, men, and their parents to bring lawsuits represented by attorneys to obtain justice and compensation and to help deter the practice.

Lay people might be concerned that the book will be difficult to read, in effect heavy going, but the book does not require any specialized knowledge of medicine. For example, it is enough to know that genital cutting can cause serious medical complications and can be fatal without needing to understand each possible complication or how it can be fatal. Nor is any knowledge of medicine required to understand that boys are not at risk of adult diseases such as penile cancer and sexually transmitted infections. Likewise, the reader does not need to know any law. American law derives from English law, which is based on plain, simple, and readily understandable principles.[7] My editors and I believe that you will find the book to be easy to read and enlightening. There are also summaries at the end of each chapter in case you want to skip one. (For example, it is useful to understand the past as a prelude to the present, but the chapter on history is long, so if you prefer you can read that chapter summary and skip the details.) You also can read the Conclusion first to get an overview of the book as it concisely summarizes every chapter.

Second, the book is aimed at those who work in the circumcision industry (physicians, nurses, medical students, hospital administrators and risk managers) or pay for it (private insurers and officials at federal and state Medicaid agencies). Hopefully, the book will persuade some of them to stop financing the industry.

Third, the book is aimed at the legal profession (legislators, prosecutors and criminal defense lawyers; personal injury, medical malpractice and defense lawyers; and especially judges). Hopefully, the book will help U.S. judges decide circumcision cases correctly, as judges in Europe are doing.

As the book is based on a law review article published in November 2020 in the *Cornell Journal of Law and Medicine,*[3] it is also intended to be a work of serious scholarship. Hence, the book includes citations to medical and legal authorities as footnotes.

WARNING! Contains sexual violence and graphic images. Like genital cutting, this book is not suitable for children. Circumcised boys and men may be unhappy to learn what physicians unlawfully took from them, and their parents may be unhappy to learn how physicians took unfair advantage of them and their son.

---

7   Riddell WR. Common Law and Common Sense. *Yale L J.* 1918;27:994. "[T]he maxims of the ancient common law … are plain and simple."
<digitalcommons.law.yale.edu/cgi/viewcontent.cgi?article=2634&context=ylj>.

This Part I asks, what facts are material or germane to the decision of whether to cut off a child's prepuce? Chapter 3 asks, is the prepuce good for health or bad for health (the American position)? Chapter 4 asks, is genital cutting bad for health or good for health (the American position). Chapter 5 asks, do people want part of their intact genitals excised without their consent?

3   Is the Prepuce Good or Bad For Health?

Before discussing male circumcision or male genital cutting (MGC), and to a lesser extent female genital cutting (FGC), it seems important to introduce the body part that male circumcision removes, the foreskin of the penis, as well as its female counterpart.

A Natural Body Part and an Essential Component of Perfect Health

The American Academy of Pediatrics and physicians in the U.S. tell parents virtually nothing about the foreskin, thus implying that it is useless piece of skin. This is analogous to dehumanizing an enemy in war. It is easier for soldiers to kill an enemy whom they have been told is worthless than to kill a fellow human being. By analogy, if parents know nothing about the foreskin, it is easy to persuade them to agree to have it cut off.

Most mammals and all primates, including humans, have a *prepuce:* in males the prepuce is the foreskin of the penis and in females it is the clitoral hood. The prepuce consists of living tissue, and it is a natural part of the body. As such, it cannot possibly be considered a birth defect that needs to be treated or removed.

By very rough estimates, perhaps 10^{20} non-human mammals have inhabited the planet with a prepuce, without suffering from genital problems, let alone serious or life-threatening problems. Most humans who have ever lived, roughly 100 billion people, likewise have lived their entire lives with their prepuce intact, without suffering from genital problems requiring its removal.

Male and female genital cutting were rare in the distant past, and they have been the exception – not the norm – throughout human history. For example, the male passengers on the Mayflower and the founding American fathers must have been genitally intact, as circumcision among Christians only began in the mid-1800s in Great Britain and around 1875 in the United States. In most countries in the developed world today, physicians do not circumcise boys at birth. Although about one-third of all males now living have been circumcised, most were because of the their parents' religion and for cultural reasons.

It is a tautology that to be in perfect physical condition, the way one was born if unafflicted by disease, and to have an anatomically complete body, a person must be bodily intact and hence also genitally intact. If any living, functional part of a person's body has been excised (or in medical terms "amputated"), including the prepuce, the person is no longer in perfect physical condition, and never will be again.

It is of course the norm in medicine for physicians to leave healthy parts of children's bodies alone, and that is the only way for children to remain in perfect health based on this common-sense conception. Physicians ordinarily only operate on a child only when the child is suffering from a medical condition such as a disease or deformity; the physician diagnoses the problem; he or she determines that the child needs the operation, and recommends it as the most conservative and optimal way to treat the medical condition. Indeed, physicians ordinarily remove or amputate part of a child's body only when it is the last resort after all efforts to save the living tissue or identifiable body part in question have failed. In accordance with that norm, most physicians in most countries leave healthy boys' and girls' genitals alone. They only cut off part of a child's genitals in the rare instance that it is medically necessary to do so. Physicians in the U.S. similarly leave healthy girls' genitals alone, with rare exceptions.

Physicians in the United States are thus outliers in cutting off the foreskin of the penises of perfectly healthy boys. You might be surprised to learn that physicians in the U.S. used to cut off parts of healthy girls' genitals as well, and no one stopped them. On rare occasions, a few physicians in the U.S. still do this today.[8]

The Prepuce Is Similar and Analogous Regardless of Gender

Both the vulva and the penis are complex, intimate body parts. Indeed, people often refer to them as "private parts" or "my privates." It is com-

---

8   Svoboda JS. Nontherapeutic Circumcision of Minors as an Ethically Problematic Form of Iatrogenic Injury. *AMA J Ethics.* 2017-08;19(8):815-24. <pubmed.ncbi.nlm.nih.gov/28846521>

mon knowledge that they are capable of giving great pleasure throughout most of a person's adolescent and adult life, so they are of manifestly great psychosexual importance. As such, among the various parts of one's body, the genitalia are widely considered to be *special,* and as being very important for a person's physical and mental health and well-being throughout life.

According to the anatomists Christopher Cold and John Taylor, the prepuce "has been present in primates for at least 65 million years, and it is likely to be over 100 million years old."[9] The foreskin and the clitoral hood are so-called homologous or analogous parts.[10] They are identical in early gestation and very similar in anatomical structure and physiology thereafter: that is, they function in much the same way, irrespective of a person's sex or gender.[11] Given these great similarities, it stands to reason that the prepuce must be treated the same way from the ethical, medical, and legal perspectives independent of sex or gender, absent a compelling reason to do otherwise.

Moreover, the rules of medical ethics and legal rules are general in nature rather than specific. For example, the ethical and legal rules applicable to heart surgery are the same as those applicable to foot surgery. It is the consensus among respected medical and legal professionals opposed to forced genital cutting that the human genitalia, including the male or female prepuce, must be treated the same way from the medical and legal perspective, regardless of sex or gender.[12] This book supports that consensus, which could be called the Unified Theory of Genital Cutting.

---

9   Cold CJ, Taylor JR. The prepuce. *BJU Int.* 1999-01;83(Suppl. 1):34-44. <cirp.org/library/anatomy/cold-taylor>.

10 See definition of "homologous." <google.com/search?q=homologous>.

11 Baskin L, et al. Development of the Human Penis and Clitoris. *Differentiation.* 2018-09/10;103:74-85. <ncbi.nlm.nih.gov/pmc/articles/PMC6234061>.

12 Earp BD, Steinfeld R. Gender and Genital Cutting: A New Paradigm. In: *Gifted Women, Fragile Men.* ALDE Group-EU Parliament; 2017-04. <researchgate.net/publication/316527677>.

THE FORESKIN IS A REMARKABLE BODY PART THAT IS VERY GOOD FOR HEALTH

Highly Erogenous

As discussed below, the prepuce in the male, the foreskin of the penis, is a remarkable part of the male body that, in its unmodified form, is very good for the health of boys and men.

The foreskin (or prepuce) is replete with blood vessels and specialized nerve endings, including "stretch receptors." The researcher Morris Sorrells and his colleagues[13] mapped the sensitivity of genitally intact and circumcised men to fine-touch pressure. They found that five locations on the intact penis that are routinely removed during circumcision have lower pressure thresholds – meaning that they are more sensitive to fine touch – than the remaining parts of the circumcised penis.

The most sensitive part of the penis is the rim at the end of the prepuce where it opens, which circumcision always removes. The next most sensitive part is the frenulum, the V-shaped structure that tethers the foreskin to the underside of the head of the penis and to the shaft. The frenulum is sometimes called the male G-spot. Circumcision removes most or all of the frenulum. The third most sensitive part of the penis is the ridged band of mucosa on the foreskin, which is analogous to the moist inner lining of some organs such as lips and eyelids. The ridged band is teeming with Meissner's corpuscles, which consist of "nerve endings responsible for transmitting the sensations of fine, discriminative touch and vibration. Meissner's corpuscles are most sensitive to low-frequency vibrations ... and can respond to skin indentations of less than 10 micrometers."[14] Thus, they are able to detect even extremely light touch. "They are distributed throughout the skin, but concentrated in areas that are particularly sensitive, such as the fingertips, palms and soles, lips, tongue, face, and genitals. ... [C]ircumcision results in the [permanent] loss of ...

---

13 Sorrells ML, Snyder JL, Reiss MD, et al. Fine-touch pressure thresholds in the adult penis. *BJU Int.* 2007-03-19;99(4):864-9. <doi.org/10.1111/j.1464-410X.2006.06685.x>.
14 Piccinin MA, Miao JH, Schwartz J. Histology, Meissner Corpuscle. In: *StatPerls*. Treasure Island (FL): StatPearls Publishing; 2012. <pubmed.ncbi.nlm.nih.gov/30085522>.

specialized erotogenic nerve endings."[15] The fourth most sensitive part of the penis is the glans or head of the penis. "The glans penis of the intact male is also more sensitive than that of the circumcised male." Thus, *the parts of the penis removed by circumcision are all more sensitive than the parts that remain thereafter.* In short, circumcision removes the most sensitive parts of the penis.

The researchers Robert Crooks and Karla Baur observed,

> During the inward motion of intercourse, the ridged mucosa, positioned now near the midpenile shaft, glides along and in contact with the vaginal wall. The Meissner's corpuscles in the crests of the ridged mucosa are stimulated by this contact and by the restraint of the frenulum, with which the ridged mucosa is continuous. In the outward motion of intercourse, the prepuce inverts (goes upside down or into the opposite position) over the distal portion of the penis (situated away from the center of the body). The Meissner's corpuscles are again stimulated, this time by contact with the corona glandis (the circumference of the base of the glans or head of the penis).[16]

Many Other Valuable Functions

When left intact, the foreskin also serves various other valuable functions or purposes.

As the physician told me when my son was born, the foreskin *protects the head of the penis throughout life,* just as the clitoral hood protects the clitoris. Even when the foreskin becomes retractable around puberty, at rest it continues to protect the head of the penis.

The parts of the foreskin – including the dartos muscle, ridged band, and frenulum – function together during manipulation and sexual inter-

15 Warren JP. Harm and physical effects of circumcision. In: Denniston GC, Hodges FM, Milos MF, eds. *Genital Autonomy: Protecting Personal Choice.* Dordrecht, Heidelberg, London, New York: Springer; 2010. <circinfo.org/Warren.html>.

16 Crooks R, Baur K. *Our Sexuality.* 5th ed. Benjamin/Cummings; 1993: p. 129. ISBN: 9780805302127.

course as part of an *interconnected system.* After circumcision, the parts are no longer interconnected.

The frenulum, which is often partially or completely removed by circumcision, appears to play an important role in *penile erection, orgasm, and ejaculation.* "When frenulum tension exceeds a certain limit, orgasm and ejaculation may be accelerated."[17] Whether circumcision removes all or some of the frenulum, it destroys or impairs those important sexual functions.

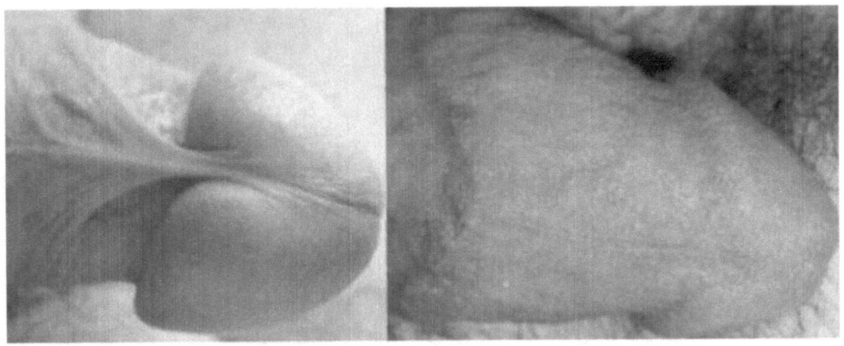

The frenulum and ridged band of the normal penis,
and the circumcised penis without them[18]

The foreskin, the frenulum, and the dartos muscle also "tether the prepuce and help return it to its anatomically correct position after deployment during erection or after manual retraction."[9] They function together to *keep the penis* straight, just as the frenulum of the tongue keeps the tongue straight. Thus, circumcised penises tend not to be as straight as intact penises.

The foreskin is highly elastic, allowing it to "evert" and "invert" – or fold and unfold – thereby enabling it to move back and forth over the glans penis and back to the base of the penis. Assisted by the dartos muscle, the foreskin *enhances mobility* over the underlying tissue.[19] After

---

17   Gentle Procedures Clinic, New Brunswick, Canada. <gentleproceduresnb.ca/penile-frenulectomy-frenuloplasty>.
18   Source of picture: <yourwholebaby.org/images-adults>.
19   Campbell. In: Alan J. Wein, ed. *Campbell-Walsh Urology.* Philadelphia: Elsevier Saunders.

circumcision, there is no foreskin left to move back and forth, assisted by the dartos muscle, as the penis evolved to do.

In addition, "[u]pon full erection, there is ample play in the penile skin to allow the glans to glide in and out of the prepuce." The foreskin therefore *provides sufficient skin and mucosa for a comfortable erection.*[20] Cutting off the foreskin can leave insufficient skin and mucosa, leading to uncomfortable erections for life.

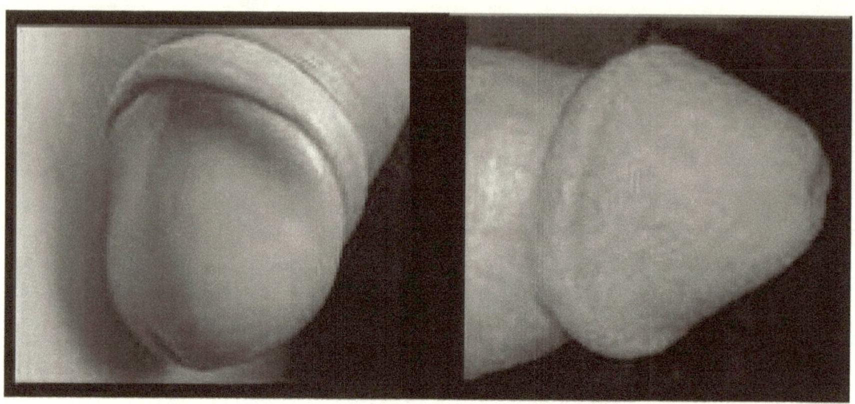

The normal moist and soft head and ridged band
of an anatomically normal penis
compared to the dry and hard glans of the circumcised penis[21]

Furthermore, like the labia minora – which serve a protective and lubricating role, are elastic, and can be manipulated during sexual activity – the penile foreskin is an elastic sheath that lubricates the head of the penis.[21] "The moist, lubricated male preputial sac provides for atraumatic [not causing injury or trauma] vaginal intercourse."[9] Researchers have established that the foreskin can move back and forth as a sheath within

---

20   Scott S. The Anatomy and Physiology of the Human Prepuce. Handout. <coloradonocirc.org/files/handouts/Anatomy_and_Physiology.pdf>.
21   Link to photograph: <google.com/search?q=moist%2Bglans%2Bpenis> Then click on "Images" if not already preselected.

the vaginal sheath in a *virtually frictionless gliding action.*[22,23] Intact America writes, "The foreskin is the candy, not the wrapper!"

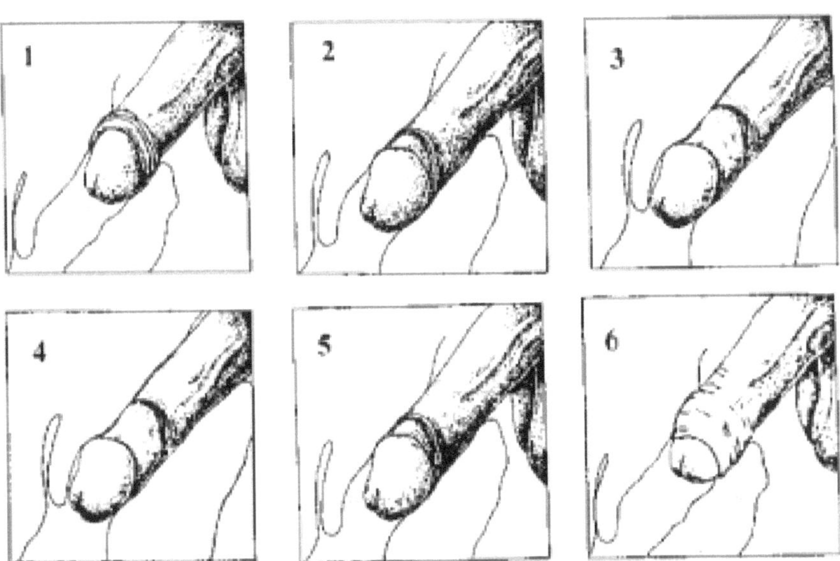

Depiction of the how the foreskin folds and unfolds in a gliding action[24]

"The outer epithelium [tissue] also has the *protective function* of internalising the glans (the clitoris and the head of the penis), thereby decreasing external irritation or contamination."[9] By contrast, circumcision turns the penile shaft and head of the penis into an external organ, which nature never intended, increasing irritation and the risk of contamination.

In addition, "[c]ircumcision removes several feet of blood vessels, including the frenular artery. This loss of the rich vascularity *interrupts the normal flow of blood* to the shaft and glans, damaging the natural blood flow of the penis."[15]

---

22 Lakshmanan S, Parkash S. Human prepuce: some aspects of structure and function. *Indian J Surg.* 1980;44:134-7. <cirp.org/library/anatomy/lakshmanan>.

23 Warren JP, Bigelow J. The case against circumcision. *Br J Sex Med.* 1994-09/10;6:6-8. <cirp.org/library/general/warren2>.

24 Doctors Opposing Circumcision. The Sexual Impact of Circumcision. 2016-05; p. 6. <doctorsopposingcircumcision.org/wp-content/uploads/2016/08/sexual-impact.pdf>.

The prepuce has *immunological properties* as well.[25,26] "[T]he Langerhans cells found on the inner penile foreskin and the vaginal mucosa, often cited as being vulnerable to HIV infection and a reason for circumcising only males, are actually the body's first immunological line of defense."[27] Perhaps research would show that the foreskin helps to protect males against HIV.

Researchers from Foregen, a biomedical company whose mission is to regenerate the foreskin, describe it as follows:

> Few parts of the human anatomy can compare to the incredibly multifaceted nature of the human foreskin. At times dismissed as 'just skin,' the adult foreskin is, in fact, a highly vascularized and densely innervated bilayer tissue [...] On average, the foreskin accounts for 51% of the total length of the penile shaft skin and serves a multitude of functions. The tissue is highly dynamic and biomechanically functions like a roller bearing; during intercourse, the foreskin 'unfolds' and glides as abrasive friction is reduced, and lubricating fluids are retained. The sensitive foreskin is considered to be the primary erogenous zone of the male penis and is divided into four subsections: inner mucosa, ridged band, frenulum, and outer foreskin; *each section contributes to a vast spectrum of sensory pleasure through the gliding action of the foreskin,* which mechanically stretches and stimulates the densely packed corpuscular receptors (emphasis added).[28]

25 Baky Fahmy MA. *Normal and Abnormal Prepuce.* Springer; 2020; pp. 65, 68-9. <link.springer.com/book/10.1007/978-3-030-37621-5>.

26 Fleiss PM, Hodges FM, Van Howe RS. Immunological Functions of the Human Prepuce. *Sex Transm Inf (London).* 1998-10;74(5):364-7. <cirp.org/library/disease/STD/fleiss3>.

27 Hammond study (citations omitted). Dr. John Warren writes, "The mucosal surface of the foreskin produces plasma cells, part of the body's defense system. They secrete antibodies and antibacterial and antiviral proteins, including lysozyme. The list of structures lost includes lymphatic vessels, apocrine glands (producing pheromones, scent signals), sebaceous glands, and Langerhans cells (another part of the defense system)." Warren J. Harm and physical effects of circumcision. <circinfo.org/Warren.html>.

28 Purpura V, et al. The development of a decellularized extracellular matrix-based biomaterial scaffold derived from human foreskin for the purpose of foreskin reconstruction in circumcised males. *J Tissue Eng.* 2018-12-22; 9. <pubmed.ncbi.nlm.nih.gov/30622692>.

- The prepuce – in the male the foreskin of the penis and in the female the clitoral hood – are natural and similar body parts, and ethical and legal rules are general. Hence, the prepuce must be treated the same way from the medical and legal perspective, irrespective of sex or gender.
- To be in perfect physical condition and anatomically complete, the way one was born, a person must have an intact prepuce.
- The prepuce is very good for physical and mental health.
- Circumcision removes the most sensitive part of the penis and diminishes sexual sensation for life.
- The foreskin also has multiple valuable functions. Among them, it protects the head of the penis for life; and as it is moist and mobile, it facilitates comfortable sexual intercourse. Circumcision irreversibly impairs or destroys those functions.

4   IS GENITAL CUTTING GOOD OR BAD FOR HEALTH?

The reader might assume, as I did when the physician offered to circumcise my son, that boys are circumcised for medical reasons. I had no idea that both male and female genital cutting began thousands of years ago, before recorded history, for reasons having nothing whatsoever to do with medicine.[29] In fact, in the ancient world, both were called genital mutilation.

VIOLENT ORIGINS

Joseph DeMeo[30] describes male genital cutting as ranging in severity. An "incision," for example, is a cut on the foreskin meant to draw blood, a nick, or a complete cutting through in a single place. In the Jewish religion, in ancient times, the mohel (the religious practitioner) would cut off only the foreskin at the end of the penis, thus leaving most of the foreskin intact. But when men tried to partially restore the foreskin of their penises by stretching the remnant foreskin (full restoration is impossible), Jewish authorities changed the practice to remove all or most of the foreskin. James E. Peron wrote in 2000,

> After performing 'milah', the cutting back of the end of the infant's foreskin, a second step, periah was then performed. Periah consists of tearing and stripping back the remaining inner mucosal lining of the foreskin from the glans and then, by use of a sharp finger nail or implement, removing all of the inner mucosal tissue, including the excising and removal of the frenulum from the underside of the glans. The objective was to insure that no part of the remaining penile skin would rest against the glans corona. If any shreds of the mucosal foreskin tissue remained, or rejoined to the underside of the glans, the

29 Dunsmuir WD, Gordon EM. The history of circumcision. *BJU Int.* 1999:83(Supp. 1):1-12. <cirp.org/library/history/dunsmuir1>. (Customary in Egypt several thousand years before 2300 BC).

30 DeMeo J. The Geography of Genital Mutilations. First International Symposium on Circumcision (1989). *The Truth Seeker.* 1989-07/08;9-13. <noharmm.org/geography.htm>.

child was to be re-circumcised. ... This is a much more radical form of circumcision.[31]

This much more extreme form is the one that is still performed in Judaism today, and it is the form that American physicians "borrowed" in the late 1800s and use in U.S. hospitals. A "subincision" in turn involves cutting open the underside of the penis to near the scrotum. "Skin stripping" is the harshest form of male genital cutting.

The prolific historian of circumcision Robert Darby, who unfortunately passed away in 2019, writes, "Even as a religious ritual, circumcision was practised by only a few tribal societies, mostly living in desert regions: the Semitic and Hamitic peoples of north and east Africa and the Middle East, and the Aboriginal people of central Australia are the most notable."[32] W.D. Dunsmuir and E.M. Gordon similarly observe that male genital cutting began among tribes in the desert belt in the Near East and sub-Saharan Africa, in tribal Africa, among the Muslim people of India and Southeast Asia, and among Australian aborigines.[29,30] From ancient times to the present, male and female genital cutting were the exception and not the norm.

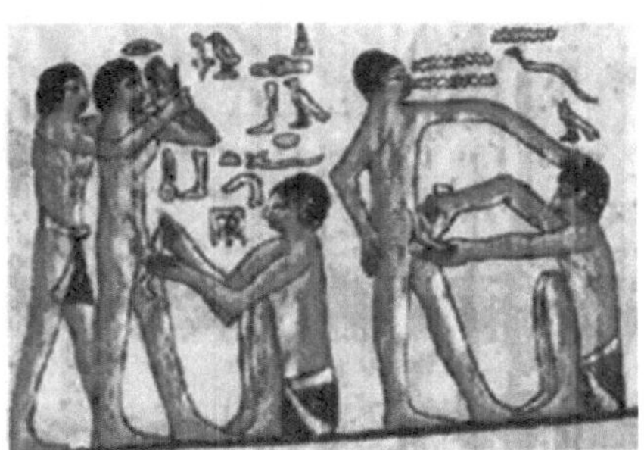

From an Egyptian tomb in about 3000 B.C., depicting circumcision.[33,34]

31 Peron JE. Circumcision: Then and Now. *Many Blessings* (Houston, TX, USA). 2000; III: 41-2. <cirp.org/library/history/peron2>.
32 Darby RJL. The masturbation taboo and the rise of routine male circumcision: a review of the historiography. *J Soc Hist.* 2003 Spring;27:737-57. <cirp.org/library/history/darby4>.
33 Offord J. Restrictions concerning Circumcision under the Romans. *Proc R Soc Med.* 1913; 6 (Sect Hist Med):102-7. <ncbi.nlm.nih.gov/pmc/articles/PMC2006243/pdf/procrsmed00871-0106.pdf>.
34 <en.wikipedia.org/wiki/File:Egyptian_Doctor_healing_laborers_on_papyrus.jpg>.

Possible Rationales

Male and female genital cutting began long before recorded history. Therefore, it is difficult to determine why people performed them. Some reasons are known, however, and the hypotheses have the ring of truth to them.

Genital cutting likely began as a *sacrificial religious ritual*[29],[23] – a "sacrifice to the gods"[23] – or an offering of a possession to the gods in the hope that one's prayers would be answered, such as for a bountiful harvest. Although genital cutting was less drastic than human sacrifice and castration, it nonetheless took something of value from a person, usually a child, by force and without consent, to benefit others in the tribe. Notably, adults did not sacrifice part of their own genitalia, but that of an infant or older child unable to refuse. As discussed below, physicians to this day target boys too young to defend themselves. (See Chapter 18, section Targeting Infants Unable to Object.)

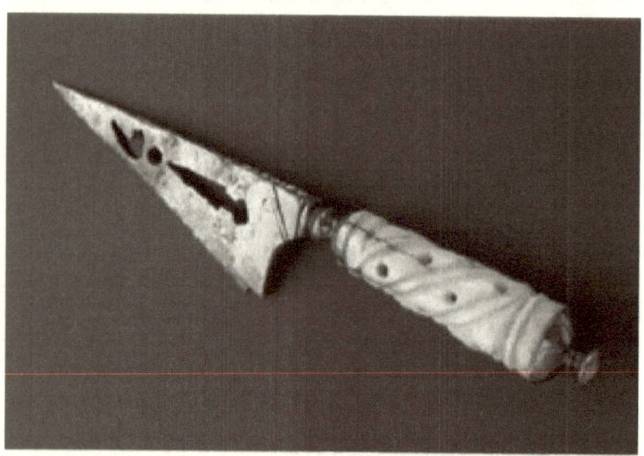

A knife used in a Jewish circumcision ceremony[35]

Dunsmuir states that the Phoenicians and Jews were largely enslaved before adopting and ritualizing circumcision. The Bible refers to the Israelites' 430 years of servitude in Egypt (Exodus 14:30).[36] Perhaps Jews

---

35 Link to photograph: <newhumanityinstitute.wordpress.com/2015/12/29/atonement-in-scripture-circumcision>.

36 Sperling SD. Were the Jews Slaves in Egypt? <reformjudaism.org/were-jews-slaves-egypt>.

adopted the practice that they had long been subjected to as a distinctive mark of being a Jew.[36] In any event, to this day, many Jews sincerely believe that their god commanded boys be circumcised on the eighth day after their birth as part of a covenant with god,[37] and that circumcision is an obligatory religious rite of cardinal importance in the Jewish religion. Jews (incidentally, my father was Jewish) and Muslims certainly have the right to believe that. The question, though, addressed in the Chapters 6 ("Adults' and Children's Rights") and 22 ("Fraudulent Legal Claims"), is whether they have the religious right to act on that belief.

Another purpose of male genital cutting was to *suppress sexuality.*[29,38] It was known in ancient times that the foreskin is erogenous or sensitive to sexual stimulation. The famous Jewish rabbi and philosopher Moses Maimonides (1135-1204) wrote that the strongest reason for circumcision is to cause pain to and weaken the sexual organ to diminish lust and sexual intercourse. "The fact that circumcision weakens the faculty of sexual excitement and sometimes perhaps diminishes pleasure is indubitable. For if at birth this member has been made to bleed and has had its covering taken away from it, it must indubitably be weakened."[39] Cutting off roughly half of the tissue of the penis does, by definition, diminish it.

In ancient Egypt, captors often mutilated warriors' penises before condemning them to slavery, an alternative to the amputation of digits and castration, which were common forms of punishment but reduced the slave's overall value. Circumcision is thus believed to have arisen in part *as a mark of defilement or slavery.*[29] Synonyms for defile include spoil, desecrate, violate, destroy, and ruin.[40]

37 Zimmermann F. Origin and Significance of the Jewish Rite of Circumcision. *Psychoanalytic Rev.* 1951;38(2):103-12. <pep-web.org/browse/document/PSAR.038.0103A>.

38 Accord FM, Thomson M. A covenant with the status quo? Male circumcision and the new BMA guidance to doctors. *J Med Ethics.* 2005;31:463-9. "Significantly, both male and female circumcision were justified in terms of managing sexuality."

39 Maimonides M. *The Guide of the Perplexed: Circumcision.* Translated by Shlomo Pines. University of Chigaco; 1963. <cirp.org/library/cultural/maimonides>.

40 Definition of "defile." <bing.com/search?q=defile>.

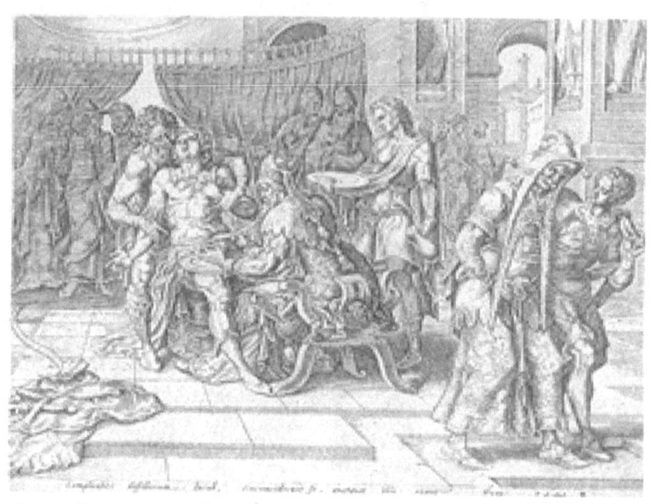

Depiction of a captured warrior being circumcised in ancient Egypt

The historians W. D. Dunsmuir and E. M. Gordon hypothesize that another rationale for male genital cutting was to intentionally mutilate and cause pain to slaves. This shows that it was known in ancient times that circumcision is harmful and extremely painful.[41] Likely some captors derived *sadistic pleasure* from causing pain to, injuring, and humiliating their captives. Today as well, members of the *Gilgal Society*[42] (Hebrew for "hill of foreskins") appear to have a sado-masochistic fetish about circumcision. One now late member of the society, who reportedly owned *The Circumcision Helpdesk,*[43] which vigorously promotes or markets circumcision [the author has not independently verified this], was convicted of possession of child pornography.

It was also a widespread custom for conquerors to bring back foreskins as trophies of war, as reported in Middle Eastern history.[44] Today as well, the Islamic State (ISIS) is reported to have performed mass forced circumcisions.[45] Conquerors do this because they believe forced circum-

---

41   Glass M. Forced circumcision of men (abridged). *J Med Ethics.* 2013;40:8.
42   See Gilgal Society. <en.intactiwiki.org/wiki/Gilgal_Society>.
43   <en.intactiwiki.org/wiki/Gilgal_Society#Circumcision_Helpdesk_-_Gilgal_Society_Rebranded>
44   Circumcision of Male Infants Research Paper, - Part Two: The History of Male Circumcision, THE QUEENSLAND LAW REFORM COMMISSION, Brisbane, Australia (Dec. 1993).
45   Assyrian International News Agency, ISIS Forcefully Circumcised Assyrian Christian Men in Mosul, Sold 700 Yazidi Women, (Apr. 18, 2014), citing *The Tunisia Daily.* There are horrific pictures of this here: <twitter.com/amirtaki/status/500190793672716288>.

cision is a terrible and a humiliating thing, not a good thing as the American medical profession would have the public believe.

In ancient Egypt,[46] male genital cutting may have been performed as a perceived *hygiene measure.*[29] Similarly, some Muslims believe that it promotes genital health and cleanliness,[47] even though running water and soap achieve the same ends.

Muslims in turn constitute the largest religious group to circumcise boys.[47] The Qur'an does not mention the practice and thus does not require it, but the Prophet Muhammad described it as a law.[48] Hence, Muslims perform male genital cutting as a quasi-religious tradition or as a *religio-cultural practice.* Circumcision is nearly universal in Muslim nations, and as a result about one-third of all males living on the planet are circumcised.[49] 92.6% of Muslim parents surveyed in a 2017 study reported that they had their son circumcised because they perceived it to be a religious requirement. Some also perceived that it has health benefits, as the American medical profession claims.[48] Given such a high circumcision rate, no doubt some parents in Muslim countries also choose it to conform to the social norm. Although Islamic sources do not set the age at which boys should be circumcised, and some are circumcised near birth, Muslim boys are usually circumcised in late childhood or in early adolescence.[48] Sarah Waldeck observed that Americans may squirm at the idea of older boys being circumcised, but in countries where circumcision is a rite of passage at puberty, people may squirm at the idea of circumcising baby boys, who may be thought as "too young" or "too fragile" to go through such a thing.[50]

46   Gollaher DL. From Ritual to Science: The Medical Transformation of Circumcision in America, *J Soc Hist.* 1994;28(1):5-36.

47   Alahmad G, Dekkers W. Bodily integrity and male circumcision: An Islamic Perspective, *J IMA.* 2012-03-09;44(1):7903. <doi.org/10.5915%2F44-1-7903>.

48   Anwer AW, et al. Reported Male Circumcision Practices in a Muslim-Majority Setting. *Biomed Res Int.* 2017-01-17. "[T]he primary reason for this centuries-old practice in Jewish and Muslim communities is religious tradition." <ncbi.nlm.nih.gov/pmc/articles/PMC5282422>.

49   Male circumcision: latest population figures revealed. University of Sydney (2016-03-08). <sydney.edu.au/news-opinion/news/2016/03/08/male-circumcision--1-in-3-globally-but-almost-universal-in-musli.html>.

50   Waldeck SE. Using Male Circumcision to Understand Social Norms as Multipliers. *U Cincinnati L Rev.* 2003 Winter;72(3):455-526. <cirp.org/library/legal/USA/waldeck1>.

Male genital cutting was performed in Africa and among Muslims as a *painful rite of passage into adulthood.*[51] It has continued for thousands of years to this day as a harsh rite of passage for boys.[52]

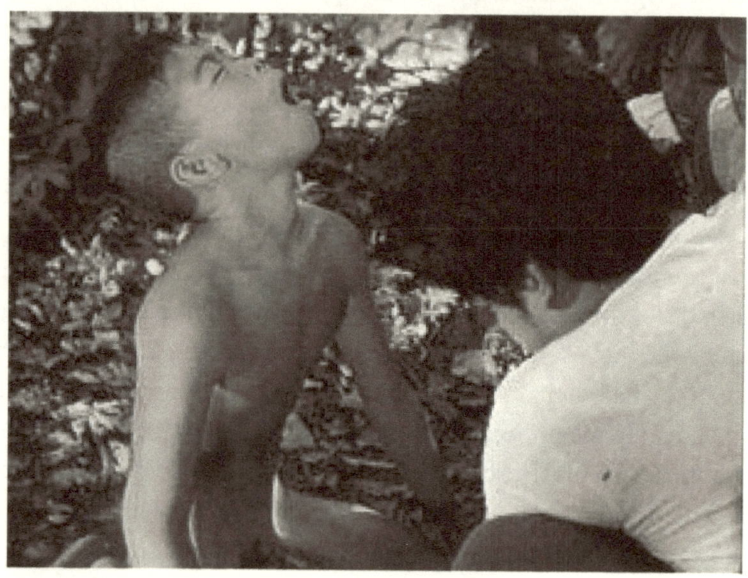

A young Filipino boy being circumcised without anesthetic[53]

Circumcision is also performed as a *mark of cultural identity* or of belonging to a certain community or class of people, like slaves in ancient Egypt or members of various religious or tribal groups.[53] This is analogous to branding cattle as proof of belonging to a rancher. In Judaism, the circumcised penis signifies that one is part of the Jewish covenant or alliance with the god of the Jews.[54] Likewise, the circumcised penis is a sign of belonging to the Muslim faith. When boys grow older and reach

---

51 Dunsmuir WD, Gordon EM. The history of circumcision. See note #29. "for Moslems and many of the tribal cultures it is performed in early adult life as a 'rite of passage', e.g., puberty or marriage."

52 McKinley JC Jr. At a Ceremony in Kenya, A Harsh Rite of Passage For a Brother and Sister. NY Times. 1996-10-05. <nytimes.com/1996/10/05/world/at-a-ceremony-in-kenya-a-harsh-rite-of-passage-for-a-brother-and-sister.html>.

53 Photograph courtesy of Medical, Cultural or 'Rite of Passage' Circumcision. *Acroposthion.* <acroposthion.com/medical-cultural-rite-of-passage-circumcision>.

54 Maimonides M. The Guide of the Perplexed: Circumcision. See note #39. "Thus everyone who is circumcised joins Abraham's covenant. This covenant imposes the obligation to believe in the unity of God."

adulthood, they may renounce their parents' religion or its practices and adopt another religion or no religion at all. Since circumcision is irreversible, however, their bodies remain indelibly marked as belonging to the Jewish or the Muslim faith.

W. D. Dunsmuir and E. M. Gordon write that the ritual was also an ancient *form of social control:* "We mark your son, who belongs to us, not to you."

Robert Darby states that although the theories about the origins of circumcision are conflicting, there is one point of agreement among these historians: "promoting good health had nothing to do with it."[55,56] In ancient times, the rate of bleeding, infection, and death from male genital cutting in unsterile settings would have been high. The practice has remained a tradition to this day among some tribes, such as the Xhosa of South Africa. When performed in such unsanitary environments by untrained practitioners, medical complications are common, and deaths occur more frequently. Among the Xhosa, dozens of boys die each year from their harsh circumcision initiation rites, with about twice as many penile amputations.[57,58]

Opposition in Ancient Times

Even thousands of years ago there was intense opposition to male and female genital cutting. The Apostle Peter described male circumcision as "a yoke upon the neck of the disciples, which neither our fathers nor we were able to bear."[59] Christ's disciple St. Paul counseled against the

55 Darby RJL. Medical history and medical practice: persistent myths about the foreskin. *Med J Australia.* 2003-03;178(4):178-9. <researchgate.net/publication/10905374>.

56 Darby RJL. The riddle of the sands: Circumcision, history, and myth. *New Zealand Med J.* 2005-07-15;118(1218). <academia.edu/9899840>.

57 Mogotlane SM, Ntlangulela JT, Ogunbanjo BGA. Mortality and morbidity among traditionally circumcised Xhosa boys in the Eastern Cape Province, South Africa. *Curationis.* 2004-05; 27(2): 57-62. <pubmed.ncbi.nlm.nih.gov/15974020>.

58 Duell M. A journey into manhood: The circumcision ceremony for teenage boys in Mandela's tribe (described by the former president as like having 'fire shooting through my veins') *Daily Mail, UK.* 2013-06-30. <dailymail.co.uk/news/article-2352015>.

59 Tushmet L. Uncircumcision. *Med Times.* 1965-06;93(6):588-93. <cirp.org/library/restoration/tushmet1>.

forced circumcision of non-Jews.[60,61] Frederick Hodges writes that "[t]he intensity with which the Greeks esteemed the prepuce was equaled by the intensity with which they deplored its ablation [removal of body tissue]."[62] The Greeks considered the circumcised penis to be shameful, something only seen in slaves and barbarians.[62] After the conquests by Alexander the Great, Greek culture and customs spread, and Hellenized Jews tried to hide the fact that they were circumcised. "Under the reign of Antiochus IV (168 BC) Hellenistic ideals, such as public nakedness at athletic games or in public baths, emerged in Judea and forced Jews to stretch their shortened foreskins with a special weight, the Pondus Judaeus, to cover the glans (I. Maccabees 1)."[63] This is an early example of circumcised men being unhappy and trying to partially restore the foreskin that was taken from them. (It is impossible to restore some of the anatomical features of the foreskin such as penile nerves and the frenulum.) The Romans in turn outlawed the practice, and violators could be sentenced to death.[33] Encyclopaedia Britannica in 1876 described male circumcision as a bodily mutilation analogous to female genital mutilation.[64] According to Catholic doctrine in the 15th century, any person who circumcises another will be eternally damned.[65] And in 1843, the Reform movement within Judaism declared the practice to be unnecessary and cruel.[66]

60   Dunn JDG. *Paul and the Mosaic Law.* 2020; p. 265. <amazon.com/dp/1725271257>.

61   Tomson P. Transformations of Post-70 Judaism. 2008; p. 120. <academia.edu/45287661>.

62   Hodges FM. The Ideal Prepuce in Ancient Greece and Rome: Male Genital Aesthetics and Their Relation to *Lipodermos,* Circumcision, Foreskin Restoration, and the *Kynodesme. Bull Hist Med.* 2001 Fall;75(3):375-405. <cirp.org/library/history/hodges2>.

63   Schultheiss D, Truss MC, Stief CG, Jonas U. Uncircumcision: A Historical Review of Preputial Restoration. *Plastic & Reconstr Surg.* 1998-06;101(7):1990-8. <cirp.org/library/restoration/schultheiss/>.

64   Cheyne TK. Definition of "circumcsion." Encyclopædia Britannica, 9th ed.

65   From Cantate Domino – Papal Bull of Pope Eugene IV. The Council of Florence (A.D. 1438-1445). 2005-03-16. "Therefore it denounces all who after that time observe circumcision ... [I]t strictly orders all who glory in the name of Christian, not to practise circumcision either before or after baptism, since ... it cannot possibly be observed without loss of eternal salvation." <web.archive.org/web/20190429233716/http://www.ewtn.com/library/councils/florence.htm#5>.

66   Circumcision in: *The Oxford Dictionary of the Jewish Religion.* Oxford University Press, New York & Oxford; 1997.

Analogous to Female Genital Cutting

There are many similarities between male and female genital cutting.

For example, there are various forms of both ranging in severity. Female genital cutting (FGC) can range from a clitoral nick to narrowing of the vaginal opening, to removal of the prepuce or clitoral hood, to partial or total removal of the external clitoris (as described in gruesome detail by the legal scholar Karen Hughes),[67] and of the labia minora.[68] FGC has been and continues to be performed in some of the same parts of the world as male genital cutting, such as in some parts of tribal Africa.

It might surprise the reader to learn that the rationales advanced for cutting girls' genitals are largely the same as those advanced for cutting boys' genitals. The World Health Organization (WHO) recounts that these include: religion; culture and tradition; a passage into adulthood; the suppression of sexuality; and the exercise of power, all resulting in social pressure to conform.[68] Similarly, a survey in Israel found that nearly one-third of parents would have preferred not to have their son circumcised, but they agreed to have it done for social reasons[69] or to conform to the societal norm.

Female genital cutting is widely condemned in the developed world, unlawful, and there is zero tolerance for it. The WHO calls female genital cutting "mutilation,"[68] and refers to it as injury to the female genital organs for non-medical reasons. The WHO states that FGC is painful, risks many immediate and long-term complications, harms all girls and women in many ways, and has no medical benefits.

As mentioned, it could be argued that FGC has the potential medical benefit of preventing the part of the genitalia removed from becoming diseased, for example, from becoming cancerous. Perhaps it also reduces urinary tract infections in girls. Richard B. Russell writes that some stu-

---

67 Hughes K. The Criminalization of Female Genital Mutilation in the United States. *J L Policy.* 1995;4(1):321-70. <brooklynworks.brooklaw.edu/cgi/viewcontent.cgi?article=1467&context=jlp>.

68 WHO. Female genital mutilation. 2022-01-21. <who.int/news-room/fact-sheets/detail/female-genital-mutilation>.

69 Ahituv N. Even in Israel, More and More Parents Choose Not to Circumcise Their Sons. *Haaretz.* 2012-06-14. <haaretz.com/2012-06-14/ty-article/even-in-israel-more-and-more-parents-choose-not-to-circumcise/0000017f-f77f-ddde-abff-ff7f1fb70000>.

dies show an association (not causal evidence) with a reduced "incidence of HIV/AIDS acquisition among women who have been cut ..." As he continues, however, "no one would advance that as a reason to cut girls' genitals."[70]

Today as well, both male and female genital cutting continue to be performed primarily for religious and cultural reasons having nothing to do with medicine.[71] The leopard has not changed its spots: whether performed on a male, a female, or an intersex child, genital cutting is still violence today regardless of gender.

VERY BAD FOR HEALTH

Extremely Painful

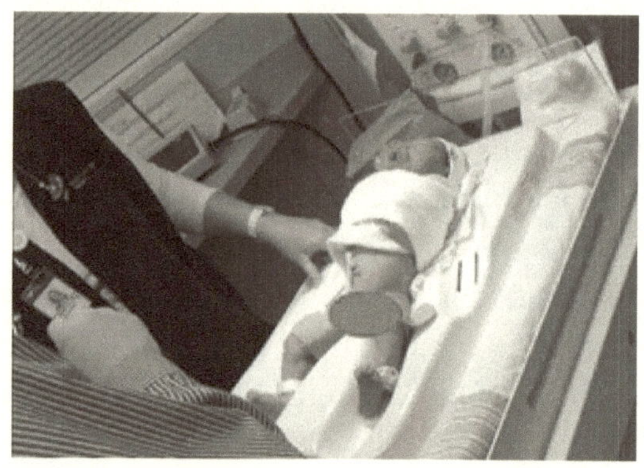

Still violence and genital mutilation after all these years

Since male genital cutting was sometimes performed as a painful rite of passage and to cause pain to captives, Jews knew that it was painful at birth,[72] and Muslims circumcised boys in part as a painful rite of passage,

70 Russell RB. Genital cutting of children as child abuse. 2010-05-18. Comment in response to American Academy of Pediatrics, Ritual Genital Cutting of Female Minors. *Pediatrics.* 2010-05;125. <publications.aap.org/pediatrics/article/125/5/1088/72431/>.

71 Freedman AL. Circumcision Debate: Beyond Benefits and Risks. *Pediatrics.* 2016-05;137(5):2. <pediatrics.aappublications.org/content/137/5/e20160594>.

72 Lewis CM, et al. Anesthesiology Transforms an Ancient Painful Ritualistic Technique into a Surgical Procedure. *Anesthesiology.* 2005-10-24;A1184. – Genital cutting does not meet the definition of surgery ("the branch of medical practice that treats injuries, diseases, and

it has been known for thousands of years that circumcision is extremely painful. Nelson Mandela, who was circumcised with the tip of a spear in a tribal ceremony, described the pain as like having "fire shooting through my veins."[58]

The physician John Harvey Kellogg advocated that children be circumcised without anesthetic so that the pain associated with it would help to prevent masturbation.[73] As it is common knowledge that the male and female genitalia are capable of giving great pleasure, it stands to reason that genital cutting can cause great pain. Until the late 19th century, physicians understood that genital cutting is painful. Common sense further suggests that physicians licensed to practice medicine would not cause unnecessary pain to children. What changed? This is a tragic story in the history of medicine.

In 1870, physicians began circumcising boys in the United States.[74] Two years later, the German anatomist Paul Emil Flechsig asserted, counterintuitively and erroneously, that infants could not feel pain because their nerves have not completely developed.[75] Laura Carpenter writes, "Many Victorian physicians embraced the perspective that infants did not feel pain. For one thing, it was convenient. Even though anesthesia became available in the 1840s, they remained risky, particularly for the very young."[76] Thus, "[a]lthough known as a painful procedure since antiquity western physicians for a variety of reasons did not use anesthesia for circumcision." Before 1978, "anesthesia was almost never used for circumcision."[72]

---

deformities by the physical removal, repair, or readjustment of organs and tissues, often involving cutting into the body"). It is also very painful even when anesthetics are used. Physicians and anesthesiologists have failed in their lengthy quest to transform violence into medicine. <asaabstracts.com/strands/asaabstracts/abstract.htm?year=2005&index=14&absnum=115>.

73 Kellogg JH. *Treatment for Self-Abuse and its Effects, Plain Facts for Old and Young.* Burlington, Iowa: F. Segner & Co. (1888); p. 295.<cirp.org/pages/whycirc.html>.

74 Voskuil D. From Genetic Cosmology to Genital Cosmetics: Origin Theories of the Righting Rites of Male Circumcision. Third Internation Symposium on Circumcision. University of Maryland, College Park, Maryland (May 22-25, 1994). <nocirc.org/symposia/third/voskuil.html>.

75 Lindley R. The Complex History of Pain: An Interview with Joanna Bourke. *George Washington University.* 2015-02-02. <historynewsnetwork.org/article/158076>.

76 Carpenter LM. If You Prick Us: Masculinity and Circumcision Pain in the United States and Canada, 1960-2000. *Wiley Online Library.* 2020-03-25. <doi.org/10.1111/1468-0424.12472>.

In 1976 and 1981, Megan Gunnar and her three colleagues showed that circumcision surgery causes a rise in serum cortisol, a marker for pain, "clear proof that infants feel the pain of circumcision."[77] In 1987, K. J. S. Anand and the physician P. R. Hickey definitively showed that in infants, the "neurochemical systems now known to be associated with pain transmission are intact and functional."[78] Anyone who performs or witnesses a circumcision can see that the child is in great pain. Marilyn Milos discusses witnessing one during her training in nursing school:

> We students filed into the newborn nursery to find a baby strapped spread-eagle to a plastic board on a counter top across the room. He was struggling against his restraints – tugging, whimpering, and then crying helplessly. ... I stroked his little head and spoke softly to him. He began to relax and was momentarily quiet. The silence was soon broken by a piercing scream – the baby's reaction to having his foreskin pinched and crushed as the doctor attached the clamp to his penis. The shriek intensified when the doctor inserted an instrument between the foreskin and the glans (head of the penis), tearing the two structures apart. The baby started shaking his head back and forth – the only part of his body free to move – as the doctor used another clamp to crush the foreskin lengthwise, which he then cut. This made the opening of the foreskin large enough to insert a circumcision instrument, the device used to protect the glans from being severed during the surgery. The baby began to gasp and choke, breathless from his shrill continuous screams. ... During the next stage of the surgery, the doctor crushed the foreskin against the circumcision instrument and then, finally, amputated it. The baby was limp, exhausted, spent.[79]

77 Gunnar MR, Fisch RO, Korsvik S, Donhowe JM. The effects of circumcision on serum cortisol and behavior. *Psychoneuroendocrinology.* 1981;6(3):269-75. <cirp.org/library/pain/gunnar>.

78 Anand KJS, Hickey PR. Pain and its effects in the human neonate and fetus. *New Engl J Med.* 1987-11-19;317(21):1321-9.<cirp.org/library/pain/anand>.

79 Milos MF. Infant Circumcision: What I Wish I'd Known. *The Truth Seeker.* 1989-07/08;1(3):3. <childrightsnurses.org/index.php/nurses-stories/circumcision-what-i-wish-id-known>.

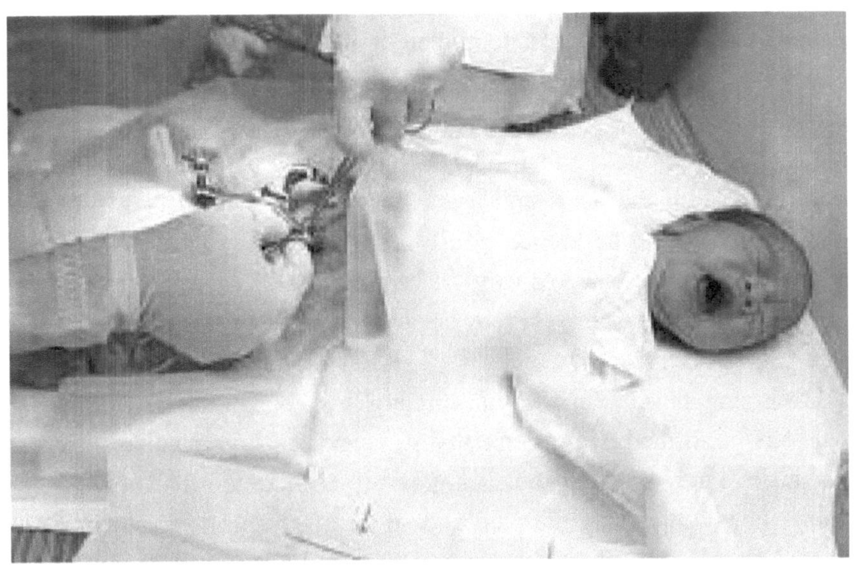

A newborn baby boy clearly in agony while being circumcised[80]

Moreover, circumcision is often performed to this day without analgesia or anesthetic.[81] It was not until 1987, or about 100 years after the practice began in the United States, that the American Academy of Pediatrics first recommended the use of anesthetics for neonates undergoing circumcision because it is painful.[82] It is dangerous to give infants general anesthesia, however – in fact it can cause anesthetic deaths, as Douglas Gairdner reported in 1949[83] – so only local anesthesia can be used.

An anesthetic cream "much touted for relief of circumcision pain," EMLA, takes 30 to 60 minutes to work, and "EMLA only relieves pain during approximately 1/3 of the procedure." It "does not penetrate deeply enough to be effective: During circumcision, the membranes are torn from the glans, the inner and outer layers are clamped, and the foreskin is cut away with a scalpel. EMLA simply cannot control the extreme deep

80 Link to photograph: <momjunction.com/articles/baby-circumcision_00398242>.
81 Boyle GJ, et al. Male circumcision: pain, trauma and psychosexual sequelae. *J Health Psychol.* 2002-05;7(3):329-43. <pubmed.ncbi.nlm.nih.gov/22114254>.
82 American Academy of Pediatrics. Neonatal Anesthesia. Policy statement 1987. *Pediatrics.* 1987-09;80(3):446. <cirp.org/library/pain/aap>.
83 Gairdner D. The Fate of The Foreskin. *Br Med J.* 1949-12-24;2:1433-7. <cirp.org/library/general/gairdner>.

pain of such physical trauma to human tissue."[84] Moreover, EMLA cream has not been approved for use during the first 30 days of life because it can cause blood disease. Another form of anesthetic, dorsal penile ring block, is more effective than EMLA, but it requires injections by needle into the base of the penis and it does not fully prevent pain. Moreover, physicians need to be trained to use it and often they have not been. In addition, the American Academy of Pediatrics calls topical and local anesthesia "relatively safe," thereby acknowledging that it is not completely safe.

Common sense suggests that circumcision is painful; any physician who has performed one can see that it is; and the American Academy of Pediatrics knew in 1989 that it is painful, as it stated that nerve block "may [not will] reduce the pain and stress of newborn circumcision."[85] Nonetheless, many physicians in the U.S. continued to circumcise boys without using any anesthetic. A 1998 study by Howard Stang and Leonard Snellman showed that only 25% of obstetricians, who perform most circumcisions, used any anesthetic.[86]

The physicians Cynthia Howard, Fred Howard, and Michael Weitzman showed that not only is pain severe during the procedure, but it continues beyond 24 hours. "Very few children receive analgesia for the post-operative pain of circumcision." Of course, infants cannot tell their parents that they are in pain, and physicians do not tell the parents that their son will be in pain, so the parents may not be aware that they are.

In 1999, the American Medical Association quoted Dr. Fred C. Valentine for the proposition that "Ordinary humanitarian sentiment prevents consideration of circumcision without anesthesia. ... I do not believe, however, that any physician would rend a mother's heart by so tormenting her babe. It is specious to hold that an infant's sensibilities are not sufficiently developed to perceive pain." But physicians in the U.S. have tormented more than one hundred million babies, often without any pain relief, without telling their parents that they will do so, and most parents

---

84 <cirp.org/library/pain>, citing Benini F, et al. Topical anesthesia during circumcision in newborn infants. *JAMA.* 1993-08-18;270(7):850-3. <cirp.org/library/pain/benini>.

85 1989 AAP Addendum to 1975 Statement. <cirp.org/library/statements/aap/#a1989>.

86 Stang HJ, Snellman LW. Circumcision Practice Patterns in the United States. *Pediatrics.* 1998-06;101(6):e5. <pediatrics.aappublications.org/content/101/6/e5.full>.

will be surprised and heartbroken to learn it. It is unconscionable to inflict great and unnecessary pain on infants, and all the more unconscionable to do so without even trying to reduce the pain.

May Cause Neurological Damage

The news about pain in circumcised infants kept getting worse. In 1997 Anna Taddio and colleagues reported that "baby boys who are circumcised with inadequate anesthesia exhibit behavior changes at six months of age that are suggestive of 'an infant analogue of post traumatic stress disorder.' "[87] In 1998, Maria Fitzgerald reported that "an infant's spinal sensory nerve cells are more excitable than an adult's. This makes their spinal reflex response to a harmful stimulus much greater and more prolonged. ... [N]ewborns have a spinal sensory system that is more sensitive than the adult system."[88] In short, infants feel pain more, and perhaps a great deal more, than adults. The Jewish rabbi and philosopher Maimonides stated, "The fact that circumcision is performed on the eighth day is due to the circumstance that all living beings are very weak and exceedingly tender when they are born, as if they were still in the womb. This is so until seven days are past."

In addition, damaged tissue can remain more touch sensitive than uninjured tissue for weeks. Worse yet, Fitzgerald found that "excessive activity (pain sensations) in the developing and still plastic neural pathways of the newborn are likely to cause permanent changes in structure." She concluded, "We and others have established that the developing nervous system is even more vulnerable to injury than in adults and that *changes to the pathways induced shortly after birth can become permanent* (emphasis added)."[88]

Wallerstein, after observing in 1985 that, "Every country, with one exception, that adopted routine neonatal nonreligious circumcision has either abandoned the practice or markedly reduced the rate of performance," stated what seems obvious: "The stress of circumcision should

87 Taddio A, et al. Effect of neonatal circumcision on pain response during subsequent routine vaccination. *The Lancet.* 1997-03-01;349(9052):599-603. <cirp.org/library/pain/taddio2>.

88 Fitzgerald M. The birth of pain. *MRC News (London).* 1998 Summer; 20-3.

be reduced [in fact, it would be eliminated] by abandoning the practice."[89]

In 2015, the American Academy of Pediatrics committee on the neonate agreed, as it stated that "[t]he prevention of pain in neonates should be the goal of all pediatricians and health care professionals who work with neonates, not only because it is ethical but also because repeated painful exposures have the potential for deleterious consequences."[90] Those consequences include the risk of neurological impairment.[91] If the AAP's committee on circumcision adhered to the guidelines and numerous warnings by the same organization's committee on pain in infancy, it would tell physicians in the U.S. to abandon the practice immediately. Thus, the AAP's committee on circumcision ignores not only medical experts and laypeople opposed to the practice, but also the warning by the AAP's own experts on pain in infancy. In short, the members of the AAP committee on circumcision do not appear to care that circumcision is painful or even that it can cause permanent neurological damage.

Risks More than 50 Complications, Some Catastrophic

As shown in Chapter 14 (The Past as Prelude to the Present), physicians in the U.S. have portrayed circumcision for the past 150 years as a simple, safe, painless, and harmless snip of a dirty and useless piece of skin, or nearly so. The author assumed that to be true, and the American public, which often refers to circumcision as a "snip," likely believes it too. But the medical profession has not told the public the truth – that it is no "snip" – and lets the American people continue to believe that it is. When my office manager's nephew was born, for example, she said cheerfully, "We snipped him!" and laughed. She and her sister had no

---

89 Wallerstein E. Circumcision: The Uniquely American Medical Enigma. *Urol Clin North Am.* 1985-02;12(1):123-32. <cirp.org/library/general/wallerstein>.

90 Prevention and Management of Procedural Pain in the Neonate: An Update, Committee on Fetus and Newborn and Section on Anesthesiology and Pain Medicine. *Pediatrics.* 2016-02;137(2).

91 Prevention and Management of Pain in the Neonate: An Update. *Pediatrics.* 2006-11;118(5):2231-41. <pediatrics.aappublications.org/content/118/5/2231.short>.

idea what had been done to the baby. One reason parents do not know is that circumcisions are performed behind closed doors.

It is general knowledge that any surgery is painful and risky. It is un-contested that newborn male circumcision risks many minor and serious complications. In 1999, the American Academy of Pediatrics itself listed the following possible complications, so it knows of them:

> ... bleeding that on rare occasions requires a transfusion; infection; recurrent phimosis [an abnormally tight foreskin]; wound separation; concealed penis; unsatisfactory cosmesis [poor cosmetic outcome] because of excess skin; skin bridges; urinary retention [inability to urinate]; meatitis and meatal stenosis [narrowing of the opening to the penis, sometimes requiring another surgery to try to repair it]; chordee [curved head of the penis]; inclusion cysts [a cavity containing a malo-dorous liquid]; retained Plastibell devices [used in some cir-cumcisions]; and rare events including scalded skin syndrome [creates blisters as if the skin had been scalded]; necrotizing fasciitis [flesh eating disease]; sepsis [potentially life-threaten-ing response to an infection]; and meningitis [infection causing swelling of the fluid surrounding the brain and spinal cord]; and major surgical problems including urethral fistula [an ab-normal hole]; amputation of a portion of the glans penis [loss of the head of the penis]; and penile necrosis [death of most or all of the cells in the penis, which may require penectomy,[92] the amputation of all or part of the penis].[93]

When the physician solicited my permission, he did not mention that cir-cumcision is painful or any of these risks. Even if he had, the disclosure would have been incomplete. The AAP did not come close to listing all possible complications in its 1999 guidelines either. The Appendix con-tains a more comprehensive list, sworn to under oath by Robert Van

---

92 Kim SD, Huh JS, Kim YJ. Necrosis of the Penis with Multiple Vessel Atherosclerosis. *World J Mens Health*. 2014-04;32(1):66-8. <ncbi.nlm.nih.gov/pmc/articles/PMC4026237>.
93 1999 AAP Statement. *Pediatrics*. 1999-03;103(3):686-93.
<cirp.org/library/statements/aap1999>.

Howe, M.D., a medical expert, in an affidavit in a circumcision case. It lists more than fifty possible complications, but the physician did not disclose a single one of them to me.

The British physician Douglas Gairdner observed in 1949, more than 70 years ago, that little was known about the hazards of the operation, and that "nowhere are these essential data assembled."[83] Shockingly, the AAP has repeatedly stated in its guidelines, most recently in 2012, that it does not know the extent of the complications.[94] It has never seriously researched them, nor has it established a central place to report the complications. Moreover, some complications occur after discharge from the hospital, and it is unlikely that the physician who performed the operation would learn of them. If physicians who perform this operation and their trade associations cared about the many types and frequency of injuries that they are routinely causing millions of boys and men, they would have set up a central database and have conducted research to learn about them. It is unconscionable that U.S. physicians and their medical-trade associations have not done so, despite having circumcised well north of 100 million boys in the U.S. since the late 1800s, according to George Denniston, M.D., president of *Doctors Opposing Circumcision.*[95]

Physicians representing pediatric medical associations in Europe put the complication rate at about 2%. Even this significantly understates the complication rate, however. According to Dr. Van Howe in his affidavit in the Appendix, complications following infant circumcisions include: infections (1% to 5%); heavy bleeding (2% to 9%); chronically inflamed tissue (5%); narrowing of the diameter of the opening of the penis (5% to 8%), which can lead to kidney failure if left untreated; and meatitis [redness at the opening of the penis that may have a sore or scab] and meatal ulceration [ulcer at the opening of the penis] *in 20% of infants* following the procedure. Given that circumcision irreversibly excises the erogenous foreskin, about half of the entire penile tissue, and turns the internal penile shaft into an external organ, the true complication rate (conceived more broadly as the rate of adverse effects) of the operation is 100%.

94   AAP Task Force on Circumcision. 2012 AAP Circumcision Policy Statement. *Pediatrics.* 2012-09;130(3):585-6. <publications.aap.org/pediatrics/article/130/3/585/30235/Circumcision-Policy-Statement>.

95   Denniston G. Email to the author.

Whether performed in unsterile conditions or in a hospital, penile surgery can also cause catastrophic complications, as newspaper headlines show. For example: "Boy loses penis in circumcision"; "3 year old Boy with haemophilia bleeds after circumcision"; "Queens Infant Disfigured in 2011 Botched Bris, Lawsuit Charges"; "Baby bleeds after circumcision, suffers seizures and dies two days later"; "Two Infants Contract Herpes Following Circumcision and Metzitzah b'Peh," [when the mohel puts his mouth on the baby's penis and sucks blood away from the wound as part of the circumcision ritual]; "$1.3 million for botched circumcision, baby had the tip of the glans amputated during his circumcision in 2007"; and "Doctor who botched 7 circumcisions gets 6 months."

In a tragic case, David Reimer was falsely diagnosed with phimosis or a tight foreskin and circumcised at six months of age. After his penis was burned beyond surgical repair during the operation, he was given estrogen and raised as a girl, but he never felt like one, and he committed suicide in 2004.[96] Similarly, in an article in the October 2021 edition of *The New Yorker,* Gary Shteyngart describes how Alex Hardy, a British man, committed suicide in 2017 after being circumcised in Canada as a young adult. "[I]n a long farewell note to his mother he wrote that 'these ever-present stimulated sensations from clothing friction are torture within themselves; they have not subsided/normalised from years of exposure.' " Shteyngart, who is Jewish, recounts how his own circumcision was botched: "The constant discomfort of a genital injury creates a covenant of pain. It is impossible to think about anything else."[97]

Attorneys for the Rights of the Child (ARC) has compiled a list of damages recovered in lawsuits and settlements arising from so-called botched circumcisions. As ARC states, however,

> This list only represents a very small percentage of the total number of circumcision-related lawsuits. Privately arranged

---

96 David Reimer, 38, Subject of the John/Joan Case. *NY Times.* 2004-05-12. <nytimes.com/2004/05/12/us/david-reimer-38-subject-of-the-john-joan-case.html>.

97 Shteyngart G. A Botched Circumcision and Its Aftermath: The constant discomfort of a genital injury creates a covenant of pain. It is impossible to think about anything else. *The New Yorker.* 2021-10-04. <newyorker.com/magazine/2021/10/11/a-botched-circumcision-and-its-aftermath>.

settlements and sealed settlements are both highly unlikely to appear in the list. Accordingly, this list grossly underestimates the number of successful circumcision-related lawsuits and the cost of male circumcision.[98]

Can Be Fatal

It will surely come as a surprise to most readers, as it did to me, that this supposedly simple and safe "procedure" can sometimes be fatal. Death can occur from hemorrhage, infection, cardiac arrest, and anesthesia. Jews knew that it could be fatal as Jewish law allows parents who have had three sons die from circumcision to leave the fourth son intact.[99] In unsterile settings thousands of years ago, the number of fatal infections and uncontrollable bleeds would have been much higher. "There must have been vast numbers of babies who died under those conditions through the centuries."[100] In the early 20th century, the medical literature also reported numerous deaths from ritual circumcisions.[101,102] The American Academy of Pediatrics has acknowledged that circumcision can be fatal when performed in a non-sterile setting.[103]

In 1949, Doctor Gairdner wrote that circumcision also can be fatal when performed in a sterile hospital setting. The AAP has never disclosed this risk in its several circumcision policy statements since 1971. Gairdner reported 16-19 deaths per year in England and Wales in the 1940s, presumably in hospitals.[83] Dan Bollinger reported a 40.4% relative higher death rate for infant males compared to infant females in the United States, "from causes that are associated with male circumcision complications, such as infection and hemorrhage," specifically during the period of "one hour after birth to hospital release (on average 2.4 days later]),

---

98 Attorneys for the Rights of the Child. Legal Victories. <arclaw.org/legal-victories>.
99 The Talmud of Babylonia: An American Translation. Translated by Jacob Neusner. 1992;251(XIII.B): Tractate Yebamot, Ch. 4-6. Program in Judaic Studies Brown University. Atlanta: Scholars Press.
100 See Circumcision Deaths.<cirp.org/library/death>.
101 Holt LE. Tuberculosis acquired through ritual circumcision. *JAMA*. 1913;LXI(2):99-102.
102 Reuben MS. Tuberculosis from ritual circumcision. *Proc NY Acad Med*. 1916-12-15;333-4.
103 AAP Task Force on Circumcision. 2012 AAP Technical Report: Male Circumcision. Pediatrics. 2012-09;130(3). <pediatrics.aappublications.org/content/pediatrics/130/3/e756.pdf>.

the time frame in which circumcisions are typically performed."[104] In 2018, Brian Earp of Yale University and colleagues undertook a retrospective analysis of all infants who underwent circumcision in an inpatient hospital setting during the first 30 days of life from 2001 to 2010. They identified two hundred early deaths during this period among 9,833,110 subjects: 1 death per 49,166 circumcisions, or approximately 1 death per 50,000. Around 1.5 million boys are circumcised per year in the U.S. Accordingly, circumcision kills on average about thirty boys per year in the United States alone.

The death rate and number of deaths are very likely underreported, however, due to fatalities occurring after discharge from the hospital that are not included in the researchers' data; death certificates listing only the immediate cause of death such as bleeding to death and overwhelming infection; and inadequate record-keeping. Yet another problem is "the natural tendency of physicians not to ascribe a poor outcome to an elective procedure," which may lead to "gross underestimates" of the frequency of life-threatening infectious complications. In other words, physicians who perform circumcisions cover up the number and magnitude of complications and the deaths.

Another study suggests a correlation between circumcision and sudden infant death syndrome (SIDS). The authors hypothesized that the stress associated with the procedure could be the cause.[105] Even if it has not been definitively proven whether or how circumcision causes SIDS, it would be better to apply the precautionary principle – better safe than sorry, – and to add the possibility that circumcision causes SIDS to the long list of reasons to abandon the practice.

The doctor did not tell me, or any parent with whom I have spoken, that if parents elect to have their newborn boy circumcised, he might *die*. The risk may be low, but it cannot be known in advance which boy or whose son will die. Whenever one does, the parents are invariably and

104 Earp BD, et al. Factors Associated With Early Deaths Following Neonatal Male Circumcision in the United States, 2001-2010. *Clin Pediatrics.* 2018-10;57(13):1532-40. <researchgate.net/publication/326040454>.

105 Elhaik E. Neonatal circumcision and prematurity are associated with sudden infant death syndrome (SIDS). *J Clin Transl Res.* 2019-01-10;4(2):136-51. <ncbi.nlm.nih.gov/pmc/articles/PMC6412606>.

understandably shocked. For example, Canadian parents were when their son bled to death 22 days after a circumcision.[106] The parents reported that they did not want the procedure performed in the first place. They acted against their instincts on medical advice, just as it was my instinct that it was a bad idea to cut off part of a penis. This is an example of parents intuitively and correctly believing that circumcision is a bad thing, only to have medical professionals falsely claim that and persuade them that it is a good thing. The Canadian Paediatric Society responded that "[c]lose follow-up in the early postcircumcision time period is critical," but physicians rarely do follow up after circumcision surgery the way they do after any other surgery. The doctor who caused the death in the Canadian case only got a "slap on the wrist." When doctors botch circumcisions, disciplinary boards in medicine mostly turn a blind eye.

If physicians told parents that circumcision can be fatal, it is reasonable to suppose that only the most religiously committed would agree to have it performed. And as mentioned, even in Israel, more and more parents are choosing not to circumcise their sons, once they learn "what's cut, how it's cut, and what the risks are."[69] Because circumcision is unnecessary, it is senseless for any boy to have died from the operation. It would be a great injustice to let more boys die, as inevitably they will, when the deaths can be easily avoided, and when physicians in most other countries do avoid them. It was a sobering moment at a gathering at Marilyn Milos's home in California during a break in a genital autonomy conference in 2010 when Kenneth McGrath – Senior Lecturer in Pathology at the Faculty of Health, Auckland University – called out the names of the dead. Of course, just as male genital cutting injures and kills boys, female genital cutting can also maim and fatally wound girls. A newspaper article from Egypt is entitled, "Girl dies during circumcision at clinic."

---

106 Dearden L. Newborn bleeds to death after doctor 'persuades' parents to have him circumcised in Canada. *The Independent.* 2015-10-27.
<independent.co.uk/life-style/health-and-families/health-news/newborn-bleeds-to-death-after-doctor-persuades-parents-to-have-him-circumcised-in-canada-a6710061.html>.

Can Cause Psychological Harm

"In medical circles, neonatal male circumcision was long assumed to be psychologically and emotionally benign."[107] As discussed above, physicians previously claimed that newborns could not feel pain, or that they would not remember it if they could, and that circumcision could never have any lasting effect on a boy or man. Tragically, these medical claims were also untrue. It is well established now that circumcision can cause long-term psychological harm.

At Birth and in Childhood

There are no randomly controlled trials showing that circumcision surgery causes post-traumatic stress disorder (PTSD) in children, but several psychologists hypothesize that it can. Ronald Goldman wrote a book calling circumcision a hidden trauma.[108] The psychologist John Rhinehart suggests that neonatal circumcision is traumatic and can result in psychological problems later in life.[109] The psychologist Anna Taddio and colleagues state that "between the ages of 3 and 6 years – the 'phallic period' of childhood development – circumcision may affect the psychological status of the child and eventually cause psychological and behavioral disturbances."[110] Yilmaz et al. have demonstrated PTSD in boys who undergo circumcision for phimosis (a tight foreskin). Furthermore, Anand and Scalzo suggest that early trauma predisposes to altered pain sensitivity, stress disorders, attention deficit disorder or hyperactivity, and self-destructive disorders.

Goldman reports how a man circumcised at age four remembers the shock and pain.[108] Another man who was circumcised at age ten, when he

107 Psychological impacts of male circumcision. Circumcision Information Research Pages, and citations therein. <cirp.org/library/psych>.

108 Goldman R. *Circumcision, The Hidden Trauma: How an American Cultural Practice Affects Infants and Ultimately Us All.* 1997-02-01; p. 101. <amazon.com/dp/0964489538>.

109 Rhinehart J. Neonatal circumcision reconsidered. *Transactional Analysis J.* 1999-07; 29(3): 215-21. <cirp.org/library/psych/rhinehart1>.

110 Yilmaz E, et al. Psychological trauma of circumcision in the phallic period could be avoided by using topical steroids. *Int J Urol.* 2003-12;10(12):651-6. <cirp.org/library/psych/yilmaz1>.

went into the hospital for treatment of a medical condition, found the experience to be too overwhelming to handle.

> I was too young. I didn't understand the effect until later in life. It made me less trusting. The terror and sadness never got processed since the event never was acknowledged. Those two things had a consequence effect on any relationship. It made me less emotionally available as a person.[108]

In Adulthood

One of the main complaints of circumcised men is that they do not like the appearance of their circumcised penis. "They frequently report avoidance of allowing others, particularly other men, to see them naked, and some, therefore, avoid sports."[15] Their complaints go well beyond that, however. Goldman writes that some men report feeling deep rage; feeling that their penis is incomplete, deformed, and maimed [it is]; and that being circumcised was the most traumatic event in their life and caused the greatest psychological damage. Others claim that it taught them how to hate; that it ruined their sex life; that they have felt unhappy about it their entire life; and that they are very angry and resentful about having their foreskin forcibly removed. Some men reported suffering their whole lives from many physical, psychological, and emotional problems stemming from the procedure. Others stated that no one had the right to cut off their foreskin without their consent; and some men felt cheated, having been robbed of what is their natural birthright (as discussed in Chapter 6 (Adults' and Children's Rights), they were cheated as having an intact body including a foreskin is a birthright).

In a 2002 article about pain, trauma, and the psychological sequelae, Boyle, Goldman, Svoboda, and Fernandez wrote, "Some studies link involuntary male circumcision with a range of negative emotions and even post-traumatic stress disorder (PTSD). Some circumcised men have described their current feelings in the language of violation, torture, mutilation and sexual assault."[81] Reasonably so, as forced genital cutting without a valid medical indication is violation, torture, mutilation, and sexual assault. (For example, "mutilation" or maiming, from the Latin *mutilus,* mean cutting off or causing injury so that a part of the body is permanently damaged, detached, or disfigured.)

Tim Hammond and Adrienne Carmack undertook a study in 2017 to document the experiences of men who consider themselves to have been harmed by circumcision. They found, as has long been known, that some men resent the loss of their foreskin; that neonatal circumcision can cause a variety of adverse long-term psychological outcomes for men; and that dissatisfaction with circumcision is a serious issue.[111] Circumcised men may regret having been circumcised and feel extremely dissatisfied that they were. Many of them find it unacceptable to have suffered, without their consent, pain, the loss of erogenous tissue, the diminution or elimination of the mobility of the foreskin, and late complications caused by circumcision. Numerous survey respondents compared their circumcisions to sexual assault (and the practice may meet the definition of "sexual assault" under state statutes).

The participants in the 2017 Hammond and Carmack study reported the following psychological and emotional harms from neonatal circumcision. To quote and paraphrase, these included: dissatisfaction with condition (77%); frustration with condition (72%); sense of having been mutilated (61%); body was violated/raped (55%); betrayed by father (50%); shame (37%); alexithymia (difficult identifying and describing feelings) (22%); suicidal thoughts (14%); recurrent nightmares about being attacked (10%); human rights were violated (73%); anger (71%); betrayed by doctor(s) (58%); betrayed by mother (55%); feeling isolated, helpless, or alone (38%); violent thoughts of retribution against perpetrator (27%); spiritual trauma (19%); betrayed by clergy/religious (10%); betrayed by tribal elder(s) (1%); other (16%) (e.g., sense of injustice, post-traumatic stress disorder symptoms, rage, despair, grief, humiliation, shock, impotency, lack of sexual desire due to mutilation, body dysmorphic disorder, deep sorrow, sense of loss, motivation to end this practice,

---

111 Hammond T, Carmack A. Long-term adverse outcomes from neonatal circumcision reported in a survey of 1,008 men: an overview of health and human rights implications. *Int J Human Rights.* 2017-02;21(2):189-218. <tandfonline.com/doi/full/10.1080/13642987.2016.1260007>.

abandonment, neglect, depression, sexual inadequacy, disgust, avoidance of intimacy, feeling cheated, incomplete, and vengeful).

Some also reported a loss of self-esteem, a more acute problem in circumcised homosexual men. There are no medical or mental health programs dedicated to helping circumcised men deal with the resulting psychological problems, which may explain why some men turn to public activism as a form of therapy to work through their anger and hopelessness. These findings were consistent with contemporary literature about the detrimental psychological impact of childhood circumcision on men's mental health. In addition, denial of loss is not uncommon in circumcised males. Circumcised males may experience the full range of distress and emotional dysfunction resulting from loss. This frequently results in circumcised fathers adamantly insisting that their son be circumcised.

In a November 2020 article, Alessandro Miani and colleagues wrote that neonatal pain and stress might carry long-term consequences on adult behavior, including altered emotional processing. "[E]arly circumcision might have an impact on adult socio-affective traits or behavior."

Some men also greatly resent having been circumcised for religious reasons. For example, a young man circumcised by a Jewish father, Eric Clopper, who worked at Harvard University, put on a one-man play at Harvard's Sanders Theatre expressing his anger.[112]

Seriously Harms All Boys and Men

I had assumed that absent complications, circumcision is not harmful, because that is how physicians in the U.S. portray it. As the physician Robert Van Howe informed me, however, that assumption is false. Pain and the loss of the foreskin constitute serious harms.

Penile Reduction Surgery

Circumcision permanently removes living tissue, of course, which constitutes a harm. It is no mere "snip" as the public perceives it to be. According to Brian Earp and colleagues, citing authorities, circumcision re-

---

112 Clopper E. Sex & Circumcision: An American Love Story. <youtu.be/FCuy163srRc>.

moves "approximately 30-50 cm^2 of densely innervated, elastic genital tissue in the adult organ"[113] As noted above, according to Foregen, circumcision removes 51% or more than half of the total length of the penile shaft skin.

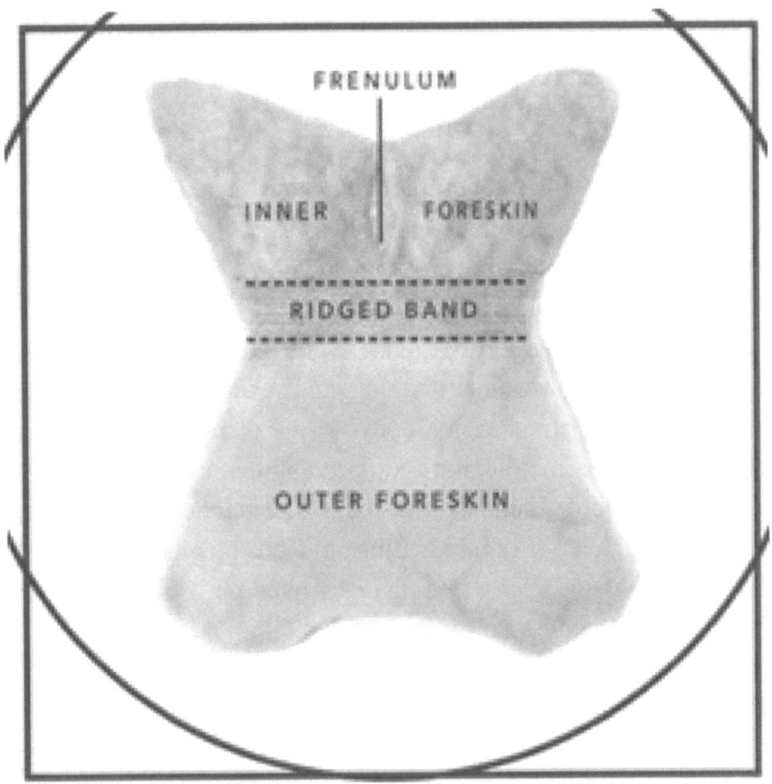

Artistic rendition of the foreskin by the Italian Vincenzo Aiello

Therefore, one adverse consequence of circumcision is that it radically and permanently changes the appearance of the penis.

As Maimonides observed, circumcision diminishes the sexual organ. One thing that the operation diminishes is the size of the penis. Dr. John Warren wrote in a 2010 article:

---

113 Earp BD. Do the benefits of male circumcision outweigh the risks? A critique of the proposed CDC guidelines. *Front Pediatr.* 2015-03-18. <frontiersin.org/articles/10.3389/fped.2015.00018/full>.

The effect of circumcision reduces flaccid penile length and width slightly, as the normal foreskin often overhangs the glans in the non-erect state. Width is reduced because of the loss of the double layer of skin covering the glans. The erect penis may also be somewhat shortened, as there may be insufficient penile skin to permit full erection. An Australian survey showed circumcised men, on average, to have erect penises 8 mm shorter than intact men.[15]

Whether flaccid or erect, then, the circumcised penis is smaller. Consequently, circumcision could also be called penile reduction surgery. It is reasonable to suppose that few men would choose to have a smaller penis if given the choice.

Warren writes, "The normal glans is an internal structure, only exposed briefly during urination, washing, and sexual arousal. Its surface is moist … However, circumcision converts the glans into an external organ." The glans becomes keratinized, meaning that its cells become filled with keratin protein filaments and die. "The epithelium [body tissue] takes on the character of skin rather than mucous membrane."[15] The color of the surface of the glans also changes over time from rose to gray, visible evidence that the penis is damaged.

Loss of Sexual Sensation and Function

Circumcisions in the United States are typically "high and tight": they remove most or all of the foreskin. Regardless, since circumcision removes thousands of nerves, which fire when stimulated, it necessarily reduces penile sensitivity.[15] Sensation may also decline with age. "Circumcised men complained significantly more often than did genitally intact men of a progressive decline in penile sensation throughout their adult years – presumably due to increasing keratinisation of the exposed glans and inner foreskin remnant in circumcised men."[81]

In addition, as previously stated, the mobile sheath of the intact penis allows the foreskin to glide back and forth over the glans. As it repeatedly folds and unfolds, the nerve endings in the glans and especially in the foreskin reciprocally stimulate each other.[15] Circumcision destroys this reciprocal stimulation and therefore it changes both the type of the sensations and their intensity during masturbation, foreplay, and sexual intercourse.

During sexual arousal in heterosexual sex, the vagina secretes lubricating fluid, allowing penetration to occur comfortably. During heterosexual intercourse, the intact penis glides in and out of its own skin sheath with each thrust. This further reduces friction between the penile skin and the vaginal wall and allows the vaginal secretions to remain on its surface. In the circumcised male, by contrast, the thrusting of the penis, which has little or no slack skin, tends to draw out the vaginal secretions and decrease lubrication. Masturbation is similarly affected: an intact man masturbates by manipulating his foreskin back and forth over his glans, whereas in a circumcised man this is not possible. Thus, a circumcised male has no ability to feel biologically natural stimulation. Circumcised males are also more likely to need to use a lubricant to permit comfortable stimulation.

To summarize the adverse physical and sexual consequences of circumcision: it removes about half of the penile covering and reduces the width and length of the penis; it irreversibly changes the appearance of the penis; it exposes the glans or head of the penis, which becomes harder and may also become less sensitive; it turns the internal part of the penis into an external organ; and it removes the most sensitive part of the penis, destroys its mobility, and diminishes natural lubrication, all of which facilitate comfortable manipulation of the penis and sexual intercourse.

According to the Circumcision Information Resources Pages, citing authorities, circumcision impairs men's sex lives. Impairments include loss of nerves and of the sensations that they produce; loss of protection; loss of the gliding action that greatly reduces friction and vaginal dryness; loss of the ability of the foreskin to stretch, which deforms the Meissner's corpuscles and produces pleasurable sensations; impotence and sexual dysfunction; premature ejaculation, inability to ejaculate, or delayed ejaculation; changed sexual behavior including masturbating more frequently, more frequent oral sex, and engaging in more risky sexual behavior.[114]

A man circumcised at age 21 for a tight foreskin (which can usually be treated by stretching and steroids) wrote, "Where I once had a sexual organ I have now been left with a numb, botched stick … My sexuality has been left in tatters." He was so devastated that he killed himself.[115] Another man described how circumcision ruined his sex life as well:

> By the time I reached 40 years old, I started losing sensitivity. It just got worse and by the time I hit 50 my penis was as numb as a broomstick. I could pinch the head and feel nothing. Intercourse was painful for my wife – she said it felt like sandpaper. I had no sensitivity, so I was rubbing the ridge of her vagina raw with every stroke, even with lube. … I was cut real tight, when I got erect my skin broke open and bled. As the years wore on it dried out completely. I explain it like this: Stick your tongue out of your mouth for five minutes and then put it back and see how calloused and dried out it feels. That's how my penis was. … Often, I'd give up before climax because it took forever. There was no sensitivity. I'd get frustrated and feel incomplete because I couldn't finish; it was like, what's the point? I just got anxious when I was having sex, and then I would be overthinking what was wrong and nothing would happen. I felt so inferior.[116]

Similarly, at a debate about circumcision, a Mexican man said that he found it impossible to understand why physicians in the United States circumcise boys. He enjoyed being genitally intact and his wife stated that she enjoyed his having a foreskin as well. He described how he taped the foreskin of his penis back to mimic being circumcised, and planned to keep it back for one month, but it was so uncomfortable to have the

114 Foreskin Sexual Function/Circumcision Sexual Dysfunction. <cirp.org/library/sex_function>.

115 Lowbridge C. "My son killed himself after circumcision." *BBC News.* 2019-04-17. <bbc.com/news/uk-england-47292307>.

116 Tsoulis-Reay A. What It's Like to Reconstruct Your Own Foreskin. *The Cut.* 2018-03-26. <thecut.com/2018/03/foreskin-restoration-retraction.html>.

sensitive head of his penis rub against his clothing that he had to abandon the experiment.[117]

Also Harms Female Sexual Partners

Maimonides opined, "It is hard for a woman with whom an uncircumcised man has had sexual intercourse to separate from him."[39] To the same effect, The *Circumcision Information and Resource Pages* states, with citations to authorities:

> The foreskin has long been known to be valuable to the female partner. The presence of the foreskin is reported to be stimulating to the female. Women are more likely to experience vaginal dryness during sex with a circumcised partner. The unnatural dryness may make coitus painful and result in abrasions. The vaginal dryness may be mistakenly attributed to female arousal disorder. O'Hara & O'Hara report that the female partner is less likely to experience orgasm when the foreskin is not present and more likely to experience orgasm or even multiple orgasms when the foreskin is present.[114]

Similarly, Morten Frisch, Morten Lindholm, and Morten Grønbæk conducted a national health survey in Denmark about the sex lives of men and their female spouses. They found that women whose spouses are circumcised reported "frequent sexual function difficulties overall, notably orgasm difficulties," and they "more often reported incomplete sexual needs fulfilment."[118]

These studies suggest, then, that heterosexual couples are more satisfied with their sex life, and therefore they are generally happier, when the male has an intact penis with a foreskin. Conversely, couples were shown

---

117 Personal recollection. Some videos of the debate are available from Attorneys for the Rights of the Child, here: <arclaw.org/debates/arc-releases-video-from-charleston-debate-victory-over-american-academy-of-pediatrics>.

118 Frisch M, Lindholm M, Grønbæk M. Male circumcision and sexual function in men and women: a survey-based, cross-sectional study in Denmark. *Int J Epidemiol.* 2011-10;40(5):1367-81. <doi.org/10.1093/ije/dyr104>.

to have a less satisfying sex life and were unhappier when the male was circumcised. Thus, heterosexual couples worldwide might well be happier if the male were not circumcised. It stands to reason that homosexual male couples might be also. Moreover, in a gay male couple, where one man has a foreskin and the other does not, their penises do not "match," and indeed they will look very different. The intact man might be happy to have a foreskin, while his partner might be unhappy not to have one and be constantly reminded of what he is missing.

CHAPTER SUMMARY

- As a court observed, it seems obvious that unnecessary surgery is painful, risky, and harmful.
- Male genital cutting is extremely painful, and it can cause neurological damage.
- It risks more than fifty physical complications, some catastrophic, including: narrowing of the urethral opening and ulceration in 17.9% of cases; bleeding (sometimes fatal); infection (sometimes fatal); loss of part or all of the head of the penis; and death.
- Since male genital cutting is painful and it removes the most sensitive part of the penis, it seriously harms all boys and men. Its actual rate of adverse events is 100%.
- It can be traumatic, and it can cause psychological harm. Increasing numbers of circumcised men are angry that a physician cut off part of their penis when they were powerless to prevent it.
- It impairs or destroys numerous valuable functions of the penis. It turns the moist and mobile penis into essentially a dry and immobile stick.
- Since it is rarely medically necessary to circumcise any boy during childhood, these risks and harms are all unnecessary too.

5 DO HEALTHY PEOPLE WANT THEIR GENITALS CUT WITHOUT THEIR CONSENT?

As discussed in the next chapter, it is a fundamental principle of medical ethics and of law that every person of sound mind has the right to autonomy, the right to make important decisions about his or her own body for himself or herself, whenever possible. Physicians, whose function is to serve their patients' medical needs, thus do not have the right to do to a patient something that the patient would not have chosen for himself or herself if given the choice and able to make it. This is the medical equivalent of the Golden Rule common to many religions: do unto others as you would have them do unto you; or as better expressed, do unto others as they would have you do unto them.

The question arises then, what would boys and girls choose for themselves if given the choice and developmentally able to make the choice? Would they choose to remain genitally intact, as physicians in most countries leave them, or to be circumcised, as is customary in the United States?

This question is somewhat rhetorical, and easily answered, by asking whether adults want to have any living tissue or healthy part of their body cut off without consenting to it, such as when they request cosmetic surgery? Of course not! People enjoy being bodily intact and they do not want to be harmed and subjected to unnecessary risks. They also prefer to make important decisions about their own bodies for themselves, rather than being told by someone else, perhaps mistakenly, what they want or what is best for them. Moreover, there is a risk that the person making the decision will act in his or her own best interests rather than in the best interests of the person whose body is being cut. That is exactly what happens when parents choose to have their son circumcised because of the parents' own preferences, such as the parents' aesthetic preference for the appearance of the circumcised penis.

As discussed in Chapter 3 (Is the Prepuce Good or Bad For Health?), an intact foreskin is an essential component of being in perfect health, and it is a body part of special psychosexual importance. The British physician Douglas Gairdner observed in 1949 that genitally intact men among his acquaintances considered it to be advantageous to have a foreskin.[83] Genitally intact men "value the prepuce's sensual nature," and reported feeling extremely satisfied with being intact. Indeed, "the more foreskin men reported having, the greater their self-reported satisfaction with their circumcision status."[83] This brings to mind the commercial where young children are asked, "Who thinks more [of an impliedly good thing] is better than less?" and they all say "more." The commercial concludes, "It's not complicated."[119]

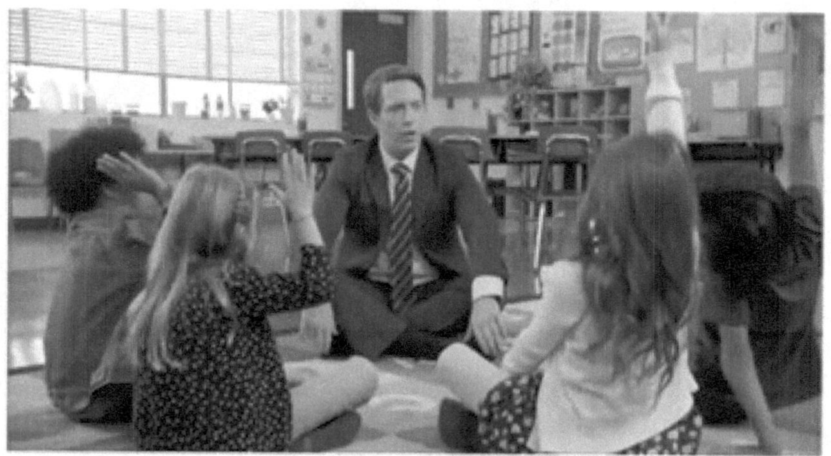

AT&T commercial. "More is better than less. It's not complicated." YouTube.[119]

Since circumcision is also painful, risky, and harmful, and as discussed in Chapter 21 (Fraudulent Medical Claim: Good For Health) it is unlikely to benefit any boy or man, we would expect that most boys would elect to remain genitally intact, and the facts bear that out.

According to the U.S. Centers for Disease Control (CDC), "[e]ven if proof existed that circumcision offered significant protection against AIDS, only 0.7% of intact men studied would agree to be circumcised." And if that small percentage of men were told the truth, namely that circumcision does not prevent AIDS, offer significant protection against AIDS, and it may not provide any protection against it at all, as discussed

119 AT&T (Commercial). It's Not Complicated. <youtu.be/gyVrvUq5PSs>.

in Chapter 21, and if told that condoms provide excellent protection from AIDS without the risks and harms of circumcision surgery, that percentage would be even lower.

Granted, some men, like some women, are not unhappy that they were circumcised in infancy, and do not believe that they have been harmed. A study by Brian Earp and colleagues at Yale University provided some preliminary evidence, however, that certain false beliefs predict increased satisfaction with male genital cutting, similar to what has been hypothesized is the case with female genital cutting.[120] For example, males may have bought into the false claim that unaltered genitalia are unclean, and they are likely unaware that they have lost sensitive and prima facie valuable tissue. If fully informed, they likely would no longer be happy that they were circumcised.

Regardless, there is no evidence that large numbers of boys in the United States *would* choose to be circumcised if given the choice and able to make it. Physicians in the U.S. who circumcise healthy boys therefore do so even the boys would not have chosen it for themselves and did not want to be circumcised. This violates the Golden Rule common to many religions, and every person's ethical and legal right to autonomy, discussed in the following chapter.

CHAPTER SUMMARY

- People enjoy being bodily intact the way they were born, and they do not want to have any living tissue or any healthy part of their body surgically removed without their consent.
- Men rarely volunteer to be circumcised; adolescent boys are often angry to learn that they were circumcised; in court cases adolescents say they do not want to be circumcised; and infants and young boys scream and try to escape from being circumcised.

---

120 Earp BD, Sardi LM, Jellison WA. False beliefs predict increased circumcision satisfaction in a sample of US American men. *Cult Health Sex.* 2018;20(8):945-59. <doi.org/10.1080/13691058.2017.1400104>.

- It can be inferred that most boys, if given the choice, would choose not to be circumcised. There is no evidence to suggest that most would want to be.
- Physicians who circumcise violate the Golden Rule and every boy's ethical and legal right to autonomy.

PART II:

WHAT ARE THE PARTIES' RIGHTS AND DUTIES?

This part discusses the parties' rights and duties. Chapter 6 discusses children's rights. Chapter 7 discusses physicians' duties. Chapter 8 discusses parents' duties and rights.

6   ADULTS' AND CHILDREN'S RIGHTS

Physicians who perform circumcisions are claiming by implication that they have the ethical and legal right to do so. Since they solicit parental permission, they are also implicitly claiming that parents have the right to elect to have their healthy son circumcised, and that they as physicians have the right to take orders from parents to do so.

These claims imply that boys do not have the right to decide the fate of the foreskin for themselves. Indeed, at a debate about circumcision in Charleston, South Carolina in 2013, Douglas Diekema of the American Academy of Pediatrics's 2012 committee on circumcision expressly stated that the American Academy of Pediatrics rejects the view that children have the right to an intact penis. He did not cite any legal authority in support of his claim. Since 1985, legal scholars who have considered the question have argued the opposite, that circumcision is unlawful and that boys have the right to decide the fate of the foreskin of their own penis for themselves.

These claims are mutually exclusive, so which of these claims is true? Who has the right to decide the fate of the foreskin, the boys who own the penis when they reach the age of consent or their parents? What are the rights and duties of boys, physicians, and the boys' parents?

To simplify this analysis, let us begin this inquiry by asking what legal rights adults have, and then by asking whether children have the same rights as adults. As will be shown, they do.

THE RIGHT TO BODILY INTEGRITY AND SELF-DETERMINATION

The principle of an individual's right to bodily integrity is foundational in many religions, "particularly the three Abrahamic religions, Judaism, Christianity, and Islam."[47] There are an estimated 1.2 billion Catholics in the world, according to the Vatican. No. 2297 of the Catholic Catechism, "Respect for bodily integrity," states in part, "Except when performed for strictly therapeutic medical reasons, directly intended amputations, mutilations, and sterilizations performed on innocent persons are against the moral law."[121] In 1999 the American Academy of Pediatrics described circumcision as the "amputation of the foreskin," and the American Medical Association called elective circumcision "non-therapeutic." Elective circumcisions are therefore directly intended, non-therapeutic amputations of healthy foreskins. As such, they are immoral according to the teachings of these major world religions.[121]

The right to bodily integrity is also a fundamental principle of "Western philosophies, such as the thoughts of Thomas Aquinas and Kant, who derived most of their ideas from Christian concepts and teachings";[121] of many countries including the United States; and of medical ethics. According to the Islamic scholars Ghiath Alahmad and Wim Dekkers, in translating "bodily integrity" to Arabic, the best words to use are *ḥurmat aljasad,* which represent the notion that the body is sacred and that transgressions against the body are forbidden.[121]

Under the Common Law

The right to bodily integrity and self-determination in the United States and other English-speaking countries derives from the common law of England. William Blackstone observed in the first chapter of his famous Commentaries on the Laws of England, "Of the Absolute Rights of Persons,"[122] published in 1753, that every individual has inalienable rights – derived from the common law of England – that are to be preserved inviolate.[122]

Blackstone wrote, *"The principal purpose of the law is to protect the right of all people to personal security.* The right of personal security consists in a person's legal and uninterrupted enjoyment of his life, his limbs, his body, his health, and his reputation" (emphasis added). A person's body is "entitled by the same natural right to security from the corporal insults of menaces, assaults, beating, and wounding; though such insults amount not to destruction of life or member," and to "[t]he preser-

---

121 Fadel P. Respect for Bodily Integrity: A Catholic Perspective on Circumcision in Catholic Hospitals. *Am J Bioeth.* 2003 Spring;3(2):1f-3f. <cirp.org/library/cultural/fadel2>.
122 Blackstone W. *Commentaries on the Law of England.* Book I, Of the Rights of Persons. Chapter I: "Of the Absolute Rights of Individuals, Parts I and II." Philadelphia: Lippincott; 1893. <oll.libertyfund.org/page/blackstone-on-the-absolute-rights-of-individuals-1753>.

vation of a man's health from such practices as may prejudice or annoy
it."

Next to personal security, Blackstone wrote, the law of England "pre-
serves the personal liberty of individuals."[122] Personal liberty is sometimes also called freedom, self-determination, or autonomy.

> Autonomy (from the ancient Greek *autos* [self] and *nomos*
> [rule or law]) can be seen as derived from Kantian moral philo-
> sophy, with key elements of liberty, the capacity to live life
> according to your own reasons and motives, and agency, the
> rational capacity for intentional action. A formulation of Kant's
> categorical imperative notes that we are obliged to act out of
> fundamental respect for other persons by virtue of their per-
> sonal autonomy.[123]

Personal security and autonomy are related concepts because individuals
who have the right to be free from harmful and unwanted intrusions into
their body also by logical extension have the freedom or autonomy to
make important decisions about their own body for themselves. Two
Islamic scholars agree that "bodily integrity has two interpretations: first,
protecting the body from others' violations, and second, the person's right
to have control over his or her body." Applying the concept of autonomy
to children, they too have the right to an intact body and self-determination when they reach adulthood.

> The principle of the child's right to an open future was first pro-
> posed by and developed further by bioethicist Dena Davis. The
> principle holds that children possess a unique class of rights
> called rights in trust-rights that they cannot yet exercise, but
> which they will be able to exercise when they reach matu-
> rity.[124]

123 Katz AL, Webb SA. AAP Committee on Bioethics. Informed Consent in Decision-Making in
Pediatric Practice. *Pediatrics*. 2016-08;138(2).
<pediatrics.aappublications.org/content/138/2/e20161485>.
124 Darby RJL. The child's right to an open future: Is the principle applicable to non-therapeutic
circumcision? *J Med Ethics*. 2013-01;39(7). <researchgate.net/publication/235386472>.

By the Ninth amendment to the U.S. Constitution, adopted in 1791, the United States adopted the entire body of British common law as it existed at that time.[125] As Abraham Lincoln famously observed in his Gettysburg Address, the United States of America was conceived in liberty, or freedom, and the right to pursue happiness however one chooses. In 1891, the United States Supreme Court in *Union Pacific Railway Company v. Botsford* affirmed the paramount importance of the common law right of personal security and freedom under U.S. law:

> No right is held more sacred, or is more carefully guarded, by the common law, than the right of every individual to the possession and control of his own person, free from all restraint or interference of others, unless by clear and unquestionable authority of law. ... 'The right to one's person may be said to be a right of complete immunity: to be let alone.'[126]

In 1977, the United States Supreme Court affirmed, citing the Magna Carta, that "Among the historic liberties so protected was a right to be free from and to obtain judicial relief, for unjustified intrusions on personal security."[127] The Supreme Judicial Court of Massachusetts has likewise observed, citing the United States Supreme Court, "There is implicit recognition in the law of the Commonwealth, as elsewhere, that a person has a strong interest in being free from nonconsensual invasion of his bodily integrity. In short, the law recognizes the individual interest in preserving 'the inviolability of his person."[128]

---

125 The Ninth Amendment to the U.S. Constitution states, "The enumeration in the Constitution, of certain rights, shall not be construed to deny or disparage others retained by the people."
126 Union Pacific Ry. Co. v. Botsford, 141 U.S. 250, 251 (1891). <scholar.google.com/scholar_case?case=12998230422916570030>.
127 Ingraham v. Wright, 430 U.S. 651 (1977) n.41, citing the 39th Article of the Magna Carta, and Blackstone W. Commentaries 1:134.
128 Superintendent of Belchertown State Sch. v. Saikewicz, 370 N.E. 2d 417 (Mass: SJC 1977). <scholar.google.com/scholar_case?case=2165107287898894579>.

Under U.S. Constitutional Law

The rights to bodily integrity and self-determination are also founding principles in the U.S. Constitution and U.S. state constitutions.[129] The Bill of Rights to the U.S. Constitution was adopted to protect individuals' rights from government interference.[130] Christine Neff writes,

> *[T]he right to bodily integrity is the cornerstone of all other liberties.* As John Stuart Mill writes,'[o]ver himself, over his own body and mind, the individual is sovereign' and '[e]ach is the proper guardian of his own health, whether bodily or mental and spiritual.' Thomas Jefferson believed that the true basis of democratic government 'is the equal right of every citizen, in his person and property, and in their management.' American constitutional and common law principles incorporate these concepts of physical liberty and bodily integrity in a wide array of legal principles, each of which affirms the central importance of a citizen's bodily integrity (emphasis added).[131]

In addition to its common law roots, the right of every individual to be free from an invasion of bodily integrity by the state has found support in the First, Fourth, Fifth, and Fourteenth Amendments of the U.S. Constitution.[132]

Thus, courts in the United States have consistently recognized that every individual has an inalienable or absolute right to an intact body, and relatedly, the right to decide its fate. This leads to the conclusion that non-therapeutic circumcision has always been unlawful, since it began in the United States in around 1875.

---

129 Mass. Const., Art. CVI.

130 Adamson v. People of State of California, 332 U.S. 46 (1947). <scholar.google.com/scholar_case?case=474434680704292554>.

131 Nefft CL. Woman, Womb, and Bodily Integrity. *Yale J L & Feminism. 1991*;3(327):327-53. <digitalcommons.law.yale.edu/cgi/viewcontent.cgi?article=1042&context=yjlf>.

132 Id. The First Amendment protects the individual's right to freedom of religion. The Fourth Amendment protects the individual's right against unlawful seizures. The Fifth Amendment guarantees that no person "shall be deprived of life, liberty, or property, without due process of law." The Fourteenth Amendment guarantees Equal Protection of the Law.

The Related Right to Personal Privacy

Although the United States Constitution does not expressly contain a right to personal privacy, the U.S. Supreme Court has ruled that the right to self-determination protections granted by the Bill of Rights also imply a constitutional right to personal privacy.[133] "These rights often relate to areas of sex, marriage, child-bearing and child rearing."[134]

Many state constitutions also expressly guarantee their citizens the right to privacy.[135] For example, Article I of the Declaration of Rights of the California Constitution provides, "All people are by nature free and independent and have inalienable rights. Among these are enjoying and defending life and liberty, acquiring, possessing, and protecting property, and pursuing and obtaining safety, happiness, and privacy." Individuals in California, including children, have "interests in making intimate personal decisions or conducting personal activities without observation, intrusion, or interference ('autonomy privacy')."[136] The court called the right to make important choices about one's own body "clearly among the most intimate and fundamental of all constitutional rights."[136]

Similarly, the Supreme Court of Montana observed that "few matters more directly implicate personal autonomy and individual privacy than medical judgments affecting one's bodily integrity and health." The court ruled that bodily autonomy is violated by a surgical operation ("invasion") imposed against a person's will. "For to say that I am sovereign

---

133 Griswold v. Connecticut, 381 U.S. 479 (1965) (the right to privacy is implied in the 1st, 3rd, 4th, 5th, and 9th Amendments).

134 Hughes K. The Criminalization of Female Genital Mutilation in the United States. See note #67; p. 349.

135 The first article of the Massachusetts Declaration of Rights (1780), subsequently annulled, provided: "All men are born free and equal, and have certain natural, essential, and unalienable rights [including] the right of enjoying and defending their lives and liberties; ... in fine, that of seeking and obtaining their safety and happiness. Equality under the law shall not be denied or abridged because of sex, race, color, creed or national origin." <https://blog.mass.gov/masslawlib/legal-history/massachusetts-declaration-of-rights-article-1/>.

136 American Academy of Pediatrics v. Lungren, 16 Cal. 4th 307 (Cal: S. Ct. 1997). <scholar.google.com/scholar_case?case=13603819742685248373>.

over my bodily territory is to say that I, and I alone, decide."[137] The court explained further,

> Indeed, medical treatment decisions are, to an extraordinary degree, intrinsically personal. It is the individual making the decision, and no one else, who lives with the pain and disease … who must undergo or forgo the treatment … [and] who, if he or she survives, must live with the results of that decision. One's health is a uniquely personal possession. The decision of how to treat that possession is of a no less personal nature.
>
> The decision can either produce or eliminate physical, psychological, and emotional ruin. It can destroy one's economic stability. It is, for some, the difference between a life of pain and a life of pleasure. It is, for others, the difference between life and death.[138]

The Supreme Judicial Court of Massachusetts similarly observed, after recognizing the individual's right to bodily integrity and self-determination:

> Of even broader import, but arising from the same regard for human dignity and self- determination, is the unwritten constitutional right of privacy found in the penumbra of specific guaranties of the Bill of Rights. … [I]t encompasses the right of a patient to preserve his or her right to privacy against unwanted infringements of bodily integrity in appropriate circumstances.[128]

---

137 Armstrong v. State, 989 P. 2d 364 (Mont., 1999), quoting philosophy professor Joel Feinberg, Harm to Self (1986). <scholar.google.com/scholar_case?case=2559844693988345859>. Professor Feinberg also has argued that children have the right to an open future.

138 Andrews v. Ballard (Tex. 1980), 498 F. Supp. 1038, 1047. The court held, "A decision to obtain or reject medical treatment is not only a personal decision, but is one which profoundly affects one's development or one's life and, as such, is a constitutional right encompassed by the right of privacy." <scholar.google.com/scholar_case?case=11956490647998889434>.

As stated, constitutional rights are inalienable or absolute, meaning that they may not be submitted to vote or taken away by the government.[139] Accordingly, any legislation that violates a person's constitutional rights is legally invalid. In addition, the Supreme Court has observed that "[c]onstitutional rights do not mature and come into being magically only when one attains the state-defined age of majority. Minors, as well as adults, are protected by the Constitution and possess constitutional rights."[140]

Therefore, every individual in the United States, including every child, has the absolute common law and constitutional right to bodily integrity, and the related right to self-determination and privacy, or the right to make important decisions about one's own body and health, by and for oneself. That is to say, the body is sacrosanct: it is too important and too private to be interfered with by any person or by the federal or state government.[141] Since male and female genital cutting both involve penetrating the body, excising healthy tissue, and are performed without the child's consent, both violate the rights of the child. Therefore, even if the federal government or a state government attempted to legalize cir-cumcision, the law would be unconstitutional and invalid.

THE RIGHT TO FREEDOM OF RELIGION

Most of the world's nations consider freedom of religion to be a funda-mental human right.[142] Freedom of religion refers to the right of every person to choose, upon reaching the age of consent, whether to practice one's parents' religion, if any, a different religion, or no religion. In the United States, the right to freedom of religion is guaranteed by the First Amendment to the Constitution: "Congress shall make no law respecting an establishment of religion, or prohibiting the free exercise thereof ..."

139 W. Va. State Bd. of Ed. v. Barnette, 319 U.S. 624 (1943). <scholar.google.com/scholar_case?case=8030119134463419441>.
140 Bellotti v. Baird, 443 U.S. 622 (1979).<scholar.google.com/scholar_case?case=13182298442826453955>.
141 Merkel R, Putzke H. After Cologne: Male Circumcision and the Law. Parental right, religious liberty or criminal assault? *J Med Ethics*. 2013-07;39(7):444-9. <arclaw.org/wp-content/uploads/Merkel-Putzke-After-Cologne-JME-2013.pdf>.
142 Davis DH. The Evolution of Religious Liberty as a Universal Human Right.

Accordingly, when boys raised in the Judaic or Islamic faiths reach the age of consent, they have the right to decide whether they want to be Jewish or Muslim or not; and if so, whether they also want to adopt circumcision as a distinctive mark of belonging to that religion or not. The chief rabbi of Israel has described circumcision as "a stamp, a seal on the body of all Jews, a seal one can never retreat from."[141] The legal scholars Merkel and Putzke observe that "the imposition of an irreversible mark of a religious membership contradicts the right to self-determination and the child's own (negative) freedom to avoid, or (positive) freedom to adopt, any particular religion."[141] Consequently, when a parent elects to circumcise a son for religious reasons, which marks him as belonging to the parent's religion, it violates the boy's and man's right to freedom of religion.

THE RIGHT TO EQUAL PROTECTION OF THE LAW

In a 1999 article, "Female Circumcision Laws and the Equal Protection Clause,"[143] Shea Lita Bond discussed how some states have passed laws making female genital cutting a statutory crime. Even a pinprick of girls' genitals violates those statutes. As discussed in Chapter 11 (Remedies Under U.S. Civil Law), any unwanted touching is also an unlawful battery, regardless of how minor the touching or intrusion into the body may be.

The Fourteenth Amendment to the United States Constitution prohibits states from enforcing laws that "deny to any person … equal protection of the laws."[144] State constitutions also contain equal protection clauses. Bond concluded in her article that state statutes that protect females from genital cutting without extending equal protection to males from genital cutting violate the constitutional guarantee that similarly situated males and females must be treated equally before the law. She reasoned that when state laws discriminate based on gender, as here, the

---

143 Bond SL. State Laws Criminalizing Female Circumcision: a Violation of the Equal Protection Clause of the Fourteenth AmendmentAmendment, 32 J. Marshall L. Rev. 353 (1999). *UIC Law Review.* 1999;32:(2)353. <repository.law.uic.edu/cgi/viewcontent.cgi?article=1579&context=lawreview>.
144 U.S.C.A. Const. Amend. XIV.

government must show an "exceedingly persuasive justification,"[143] which it cannot do. Bond observed that male and female genital cutting both inflict serious pain; both risk complications, some severe, and death; and both seriously harm their victims.[145] She concluded that states must either strike down the state statutes protecting girls as unconstitutional or extend equal protection to boys.[145,146]

In California, for example, one statute protects girls from non-therapeutic genital cutting, while another statute prohibits cities from restricting male genital cutting. These conflicting laws violate the Equal Protection Clauses of the United States and California constitutions.

Physicians are also ethically proscribed from discriminating between the male and female genitalia without a compelling medical justification. AMA Code of Medical Ethics Opinion 1.1.2. Prospective Patients, explains that physicians "may not discriminate against a patient on the basis of gender identity, sexual orientation, or other nonclinical characteristics."[147]

CHILDREN ALSO HAVE THE SAME RIGHTS UNDER INTERNATIONAL LAW

As discussed below, children also have comparable rights under international law.

Several United Nations documents together form the International Bill of Rights,[148] and most countries have ratified them as treaties and have thereby voluntarily accepted them as binding. Article VI, Section 2 of the

---

145 Id. at n. 100.
146 See also: Povennmire R. Do Parents Have the Legal Authority to Consent to the Surgical Amputation of Normal, Healthy Tissue From Their Infant Children? *Am Univ J Gend Soc Policy Law.* 1998-99;7(1):87-123. "Overbroad distinctions between 'genital mutilation' and 'circumcision' cannot obscure the unconstitutional and discriminatory effect of the Anti-FGM Act." <digitalcommons.wcl.american.edu/cgi/viewcontent.cgi?referer&<httpsredir=1&article=1192&context=jgspl>.
147 Hahn Chaet D. AMA Code of Medical Ethics' Opinions Related to Discrimination and Disparities in Health Care. *AMA J Ethics.* 2016-11. <journalofethics.ama-assn.org/article/ama-code-medical-ethics-opinions-related-discrimination-and-disparities-health-care/2016-11>.
148 The Office of the United Nations High Commissioner for Human Rights sets out the treaties comprising the International Bill of Rights, and the core international human rights treaties and documents. <ohchr.org/en/instruments-and-mechanisms/international-human-rights-law>.

United States Constitution provides that such treaties are the supreme law of the land.

The right to bodily integrity and self-determination is recognized by all democratic countries and codified in some of their constitutions. The 1948 Universal Declaration of Human Rights recognizes every person's right to life and liberty as a fundamental principle of international law as well, and indeed it is a universal human right.[149,150] As Svoboda writes, "human rights protect the bodily integrity of all infants against any unnecessary and non-medically indicated intrusion."[151] Similarly, under European law applicable to all European nations, "Everyone has the right to liberty and security of the person."

The United Nations Charter requires member states to promote human rights and fundamental freedoms without distinction as to race, sex, or religion.[152] The Charter specifies that children have the same human rights as adults, and special rights arising from their need for special protection during their minority. The 1948 Universal Declaration of Human Rights recognizes every person's right to freedom from cruel or degrading treatment.[153] The 1989 Convention on the Rights of the Child establishes customary international law applicable to children worldwide, even though the United States has not ratified it. Article 3 thereof requires that member states' legal institutions make their primary consideration the best interests of the child, and ensure the child such protection and care as is necessary for his or her well-being. Article 6 recognizes that every child has the inherent right to life. Article 19 recognizes children's rights to special protection from mental or physical violence or abuse by parents or anyone caring for the child. Article 24.3 requires abolishing traditional practices prejudicial to the health of children. Article 34 protects children from sexual abuse. Article 36 protects children from exploitation prejudicial to the child's welfare. The 1996 International Covenant on Civil

---

149 GW. [Constitution] Art. 11 (Neth.) "Everyone shall have the right to inviolability of his person, without prejudice to restrictions laid down by or pursuant to Act of Parliament.

150 Eur. Conv. on H.R. (following T3.4 – BAS) Art. 5(1) "Everyone has the right to liberty and security of the person."

151 Svoboda JS. Circumcision of male infants as a human rights violation. *J Med Ethics.* 2013;39;469-74.

152 UN Charter, Preamble and Article 56.

153 Id., Art. 5.

and Political Rights also gives minors the right to protection from family, society, and the state.[154] Non-therapeutic, non-consensual genital cutting, whether of boys or of girls, violates every one of these provisions of international law.

The Royal Dutch Medical Association,[155] the South African Medical Association,[156] the Tasmania Law Reform Institute,[157] the Slovenian human rights ombudsman,[158] and the Norwegian ombudsman[159] have all concluded that male circumcision constitutes a human rights violation. In an article published by the Netherlands Institute of Human Rights, Jacqueline Smith wrote,

> The focus must be placed on the children who are forced to suffer without consent. Male circumcision is, like female genital mutilation, a 'harmful traditional practice' and as such is in violation with the [international] rights of the child. It is necessary to advocate full respect for these human rights for all children, boys and girls alike.[160]

The British Medical Association has also observed that if circumcision is prejudicial to a child's health and well-being, meaning if it is risky and/or

---

154 Id., Art. 24.

155 The Royal Dutch Medical Association circumcision policy statement (2010) (adopting a policy of strong deterrence due in part to the increasing emphasis on children's rights).

156 Friedman J. South African Medical Association denounces circumcision of infants, (denouncing male infant circumcision as "unethical" and "illegal"). *Attorneys for the Rights of the Child Newsletter.* 2011-06-26;9(1). <nocirc-sa.co.za/in-the-news/south-african-medical-association-sama-denounces-circumcision-of-infants>.

157 Tasmania Law Reform Inst. Non-therapeutic Male Circumcision. Issues Paper #14. 2009-06;4.

158 Slovenian human rights ombudsman. [Circumcision of boys for non-medical reasons is a violation of children's rights] (Original in Slovenian). 2012-02-03. <varuh-rs.si/sl/obravnavane-pobude/primer/obrezovanje-fantkov-iz-nemedicinskih-razlogov-je-krsitev-otrokovih-pravic/>.

159 Norway: Ombudsman proposes setting minimum age for male circumcision. *Child Rights Int Network* (CRIN). 2011-02-09. Norway's ombudsman proposed a minimum age of 15 or 16 for ritual male circumcision to respect children's best interests and their right to self-determination on religious and health matters. <archive.crin.org/en/library/news-archive/norway-ombudsman-proposes-setting-minimum-age-male-circumcision.html>.

160 Smith J. Male Circumcision and the Rights of the Child. In: Bulterman M, Hendriks A, Smith J (eds.). *To Baehr in Our Minds: Essays in Human Rights from the Heart of the Netherlands.* Netherlands Inst of Human Rights (SIM), Univ. Utrecht, Netherlands. 1998;465-98. <cirp.org/library/legal/smith>.

harmful – which it is – it is likely that a legal challenge on human rights grounds will be successful.[161]

Thus, the unnecessary genital cutting of minors violates numerous provisions of international law and the human rights of every child in every country in the world.

CHAPTER SUMMARY

- Unnecessary genital cutting violates the inalienable or absolute rights of the child to personal security or bodily integrity; to self-determination or freedom or autonomy, the right to pursue happiness however one chooses; and to privacy.
- Unnecessary genital cutting for religious reasons violates the child's right to freedom of religion.
- Male genital cutting also violates the constitutional right of males to Equal Protection of the Law, as females are protected from unnecessary genital cutting.
- Male and female genital cutting also violate international law and constitute a human rights violation.

In short, it is unlawful under numerous provisions of United States law, the common law, the laws of many countries, and international law, including human rights law, for physicians to cut the genitals of any healthy boy or girl.

---

161 British Medical Association, Medical Ethics Commitee. The law & ethics of male circumcision – guidance for doctors. 2003-04-04. <cirp.org/library/statements/bma2003>.

7 PHYSICIANS' DUTIES

This chapter asks, what duties do physicians have to their patients, and are physicians allowed to circumcise healthy boys? If they are not allowed to do so, it will follow that they are not allowed to solicit parental permission for the operation either.

COMPLY WITH THE LAW AND THE RULES OF MEDICAL ETHICS

Of course, every person and legal entity in the United States has a duty to obey the law. Those who violate civil laws can be held liable in a civil court for monetary damages, while those who violate the criminal law can be prosecuted by the state and punished through fines and/or imprisonment. Since medicine involves life and death decisions, it is particularly important that medical professionals, hospitals, and medical associations be familiar with and adhere to laws applicable to the practice of medicine. Medical associations are well-financed, they have in-house counsel, and they have the resources to hire the best law firms in the country. The American Academy of Pediatrics even had a lawyer on the committee that issued circumcision guidelines in 2012. If anyone should know the law, physicians and their hospitals and medical associations should know the law, given the potentially dire ramifications of disobeying it. In any event, it is a fundamental legal principle that ignorance is no excuse for breaking a law.

When physicians become licensed to practice medicine in the United States, they also become subject to the ethical or moral rules of conduct promulgated by the American Medical Association in the Code of Medical Ethics, which date back to 1847.[162] The Code states that these ethical rules exist primarily for the benefit of the patient.[163] "A physician's violation of an ethical duty is a serious matter that can result in reprimand

---

162 Reddick FA Jr. The Code of Medical Ethics of the American Medical Association. *Ochsner J.* 2003 Spring;5(2):6-10. <ncbi.nlm.nih.gov/pmc/articles/PMC3399321>.

163 AMA Principles of Medical Ethics, Preamble. <ama-assn.org/about/publications-newsletters/ama-principles-medical-ethics>.

by a board of licensure, suspension of the physician's license to practice medicine, or even revocation of the right to practice medicine."[164]

When Felix Daase was a law student of mine, he hypothesized that the legal and ethical rules governing the practice of medicine would be identical. This was a brilliant insight, and we found that to be the case. As one example, physicians have an ethical duty to obey the law as well as a legal duty to do so. Principle I of the AMA Code of Medical Ethics provides that "A physician shall … respect human dignity and rights."[163] Principle III provides, "A physician shall respect the law and also recognize a responsibility to seek changes in those requirements which are contrary to the best interests of the patient." Principle IV states, "A physician shall respect the rights of patients."[163]

Because physicians have a duty to respect the legal right of every individual to bodily integrity, self-determination, and privacy, they have a duty to discharge patients they pronounce healthy and bodily intact. The parallel ethical duty is the rule of "nonmaleficence," enumerated by Beauchamp and Childress in 2008. It is embodied by the Hippocratic Oath that medical students swear to abide by when they become doctors: "First, Do No Harm." Physicians who circumcise take healthy boys and seriously harm them in violation of the Hippocratic Oath.

Physicians also have a duty to respect the related legal right of individuals to self-determination.[165] The parallel ethical duty is the rule of autonomy. The Code of Medical Ethics provides that "Respect for patient autonomy is central to professional ethics."[166] The human rights attorney Steven Svoboda calls patient autonomy "perhaps the paramount ethical

164 Hafemeister TL, Gulbrandsen RM Jr. The Fiduciary Obligation of Physicians to "Just Say No" If an "Informed" Patient Demands Services that Are Not Medically Indicated. *Seton Hall L Rev.* 2009-04-06;39(2):335-86, p. 383. <scholarship.shu.edu/cgi/viewcontent.cgi?article=1010&context=shlr>.

165 In Schloendorff v. Society of New York Hospital in 1914, Justice Benjamin Cardozo of the New York Court of Appeals famously wrote: "Every human being of adult years and sound mind has a right to determine what shall be done with his own body; and a surgeon who performs an operation without his patient's consent commits an assault for which he is liable in damages. This is true except in cases of emergency where the patient is unconscious and where it is necessary to operate before consent can be obtained." Cited in Matter of Conroy, 486 A. 2d 1209 (NJ: Supreme Court 1985). <scholar.google.com/scholar_case?case=2290154573715145215>.

166 Opinion 2.2.1, AMA Code of Medical Ethics. <ama-assn.org/system/files/2019-06/code-of-medical-ethics-chapter-2.pdf>.

principle in Western medicine."[8] (Although cosmetic surgery intrudes into the body and constitutes an assault, the assault is legally permitted because the adult on whom the operation is being performed has requested it and consented to it.)

Since unnecessary surgery is harmful, it is unethical when performed without fully informed adult consent. It is also unlawful. As a California court observed in 2006 in *Tortorella v. Castro,* where a physician subjected an adult to unnecessary surgery, it seems obvious that it is inherently injurious or harmful to needlessly go under the knife.[167] It causes unnecessary pain and suffering; it unnecessarily risks complications; it is harmful to remove healthy tissue and a functional body part; and it leaves a scar as evidence of a wound. The court held that unnecessary surgery is unlawful and that physicians are liable for the resulting harm that it causes. Similarly, Massachusetts regulations in the context of worker's compensation claims provide that unnecessary surgery is an abuse of the license to practice medicine.[168]

ACT IN THE BEST INTERESTS OF EACH PATIENT

As courts have observed, physicians have superior knowledge of medicine and experience vis-à-vis their patients, and they have dominant bargaining power: "the players are on unequal playing fields."[169] (I certainly sensed that when the physician solicited my permission. As mentioned, I thought of him as a world expert on circumcision, whereas I knew nothing about it. In fact, what I believed, that it was a painless, harmless snip of a useless piece of skin, was false.) Anyone undergoing any surgery knows that the physician has superior knowledge of medicine. Physicians have the power to use their medical training to heal patients or to preserve their health, but they also have the power to destroy or to end a patient's life. Patients in turn, who know little or nothing

---

167 Tortorella v. Castro, 140 Cal. Rptr. 3d. 853 (Cal. 2006). <scholar.google.com/scholar_case?case=8009703171466596993>.

168 Massachusetts Workers' Compensation Advisory Council. *FY '16 Annual Report.* 2017-06-12; p. 94.<mass.gov/files/documents/2017/10/05/wcac-2016-annual-report.pdf>.

169 Thierfelder v. Wolfert, 52 A. 3d 1251, 1260 (Pa: S. Ct. 2012). <scholar.google.com/scholar_case?case=2815705820590279872>.

about medicine, have no choice but to trust physicians with their health and safety. It is incumbent on courts to protect trusting patients from malfeasance by medical professionals.[169]

Children who have developed enough to be able to reason are even more vulnerable than adults, and they can be easily persuaded to consent to a medical procedure by physicians and parents, while newborn boys literally know nothing and are completely vulnerable. Courts therefore impose upon physicians a strict fiduciary duty, the highest duty in the law,[170] to act in the best interests of each patient, keeping the patient's best interests and health and welfare at the forefront.[171] Physicians have a parallel ethical duty to do what is best for the patient's welfare under the Code of Medical Ethics: "The patient should ... be able to trust [that] the physician will act in the [patient's] best interests."[172] The case law and rules of medical ethics set forth numerous subsidiary fiduciary duties that physicians owe their patients as discussed below.

JUSTIFY EVERY MEDICAL PROCEDURE ON MEDICAL GROUNDS

Physicians are only licensed to practice medicine. As the Code of Medical Ethics states, their function is to provide competent medical care,[173] to serve their patients' medical needs,[174] and to help alleviate their patients' suffering.[174] As a result, physicians have an ethical[164] and a legal[175,176,177] duty to justify every medical intervention on medical grounds.

170 "In fact, there is no higher standard of care than a fiduciary duty." <thinkeenlegal.com/2016/12/28/ex-fide-fiducia-physicians-fiduciary-duties-according-to-the-doj>.

171 "The patient should ... be able to trust [that] the physician will act in the [patient's] best interests." <casetext.com/case/petrillo-v-syntex-laboratories-inc>

172 Similarly, Article VIII of the AMA Code of Medical Ethics provides, "A physician shall, while caring for a patient, regard responsibility to the patient as paramount." The "best interests" of the child is also a guiding principle of the Convention on the Rights of the Child. <un.org/womenwatch/daw/csw/csw52/statements_missions/Interagency_Statement_on_Eliminating_FGM.pdf>.

173 AMA Code of Medical Ethics, Principle I.

174 AMA Code of Medical Ethics, Opinion 1.1.1. "A patient-physician relationship exists when a physician serves a patient's medical needs." <ama-assn.org/system/files/code-of-medical-ethics-chapter-1.pdf>.

175 AMA Code of Medical Ethics, Principle I. "A physician shall be dedicated to providing competent medical care." <ama-assn.org/about/publications-newsletters/ama-principles-medical-ethics>.

The British Medical Association acknowledges this in the context of male circumcision: "As with any other aspect of care, health care professionals must be able to justify their decisions …"[178] Thirty-eight medical experts representing pediatric medical associations in Northern Europe agree in an article about circumcision: "It is commonly accepted that medical procedures always need to be justified because of their invasive nature and possible damaging effects." As to preventive medical procedures, the European experts continue,

> Preventive medical procedures need more and stricter justification than do therapeutic medical procedures, as they are aimed at people who are generally free of medical problems. Even stricter criteria apply for preventive medical procedures in children, who cannot weigh the evidence themselves and cannot legally consent to the procedure.[179] …
>
> Physicians are well-educated, well-trained professionals who are and should be responsible for determining whether a requested course of treatment is medically appropriate. … *[Physicians] must appraise whether a requested treatment is medically indicated for a given patient.* … The physician is not a subservient pawn in the patient's life, but an erudite and trustworthy partner dedicated to promoting and protecting a patient's medical well-being.[179]

---

176 AMA Code of Medical Ethics, Opinion 1.1.1. Physicians have a duty "to use sound medical judgment on patients' behalf." See note #174.

177 AMA Code of Medical Ethics, Opinion 1.1.6. "physicians individually and collectively share the obligation to ensure that the care patients receive is safe, effective, patient centered, timely, efficient, and equitable." See note #174.

178 British Medical Association. Non-therapeutic male circumcision (NTMC) of children – practical guidance for doctors. BMA circumcision policy statement. 2019; p. 17. <bma.org.uk/media/1847/bma-non-therapeutic-male-circumcision-of-children-guidance-2019.pdf>.

179 Frisch M, et al. Cultural Bias in the AAP's 2012 Technical Report and Policy Statement on Male Circumcision, citing Consent, Rights and Choices in Health Care for Children and Young People. BMA Ethics Committee. London, UK: BMJ Books, Wiley; 2000. *Pediatrics.* 2013-04;131(4):796-800 at 2. <pediatrics.aappublications.org/content/131/4/796>.

A medical dictionary gives two definitions of "indicate."[180] One is a sign or symptom of a medical condition requiring treatment, for example, "the high fever indicates a serious condition." The other is, "to demonstrate or suggest the necessity or advisability of," e.g., the "indicated treatment" for a medical condition. Therefore, surgery is only medically indicated when a physician determines that the surgery is *medically necessary and advisable,* in the independent medical judgment of the physician, to treat a patient suffering from a medical condition.

Even when a treatment is medically indicated, physicians must diagnose the medical condition and consider the "effectiveness of appropriate medical therapies and the needs and interests of the patient."[181] The Supreme Court of California also has observed[182] that a physician has a duty to explore treatment alternatives. The Code of Medical Ethics similarly states in the context of minors that physicians must, "[b]ase recommendations for treatment on the likely benefit to the patient, taking into account the effectiveness of treatment, risks of additional suffering with and without treatment, available alternatives, and overall prognosis."[181] After all, why should a patient be subjected to a treatment if the outcome will be the same or better if the physician does nothing? Patients have the right, "to expect that their physicians will provide guidance about what they consider the optimal course of action for the patient [that is, each and every patient] *based on the physician's objective professional judgment*" (emphasis added).[183] Thus, a physician has a duty to disregard what parents want, and to reject what American medical association say in their circumcision guidelines, if different from what the physician determines is best for the patient. Importantly, then, physicians are not allowed to rely upon and hide behind medical association guidelines that are inconsistent with what they would recommend for each child using their independent objective medical judgment.

---

180 Definition of "indicated." <merriam-webster.com/dictionary/indicated>.
181 AMA Code of Medical Ethics, Principle 2.2.1: Pediatric Decision Making. <ama-assn.org/delivering-care/ethics/pediatric-decision-making>.
182 Arato v. Avedon, 13 Cal. App. 4th 1172, 858 P.2d 598 (1993). <scholar.google.com/scholar_case?case=14162459049776572406>.
183 AMA Code of Medical Ethics, Opinion 1.1.3, Patient Rights. See note #174.

OBTAIN THE PATIENT'S FULLY INFORMED CONSENT WHENEVER POSSIBLE

Katz and Webb write, "The current concept of informed consent in medical practice has roots within both ethical theory and law. The support for informed consent in ethical theory is most commonly found in the concept of autonomy, the right of an autonomous agent to make decisions as guided by his or her own reason."[184] In *Arato v. Avedon,* [182] a California court stated that a physician has, "a fiduciary duty to a patient to make a full and fair disclosure to the patient of all facts which materially affect the patient's rights and interests," so that the patient will be able to make an informed decision about a recommended medical procedure.[182] In *Cobbs v. Grant,* the court held that physicians have a duty to disclose therapeutic alternatives and their hazards.[185] Similarly, in *Moore v. Regents of University of California,* the Supreme Court of California stated that "in soliciting the patient's consent, *a physician has a fiduciary duty to disclose all information material to the patient's decision* (emphasis added)."[186] In short, physicians must disclose anything and everything that might affect the decision by the patient or the patient's proxy.

Likewise, the AMA Code of Medical Ethics requires that physicians inform the patient about the diagnosis of his or her medical condition, the nature and purpose of recommended interventions, and the burdens, risks, and expected benefits of all options, including the option of forgoing treatment.[187] Physicians also must respect the patient's right to refuse a recommended treatment.[188] "Without fully informed consent, the treatment constitutes a battery."[189]

184 Katz AL, Webb SA. Informed Consent in Decision-Making in Pediatric Practice. *Pediatrics.* 2016-08;138(2). <pediatrics.aappublications.org/content/138/2/e20161485>.

185 Cobbs v. Grant, 83 Cal. 3d 229, 243-43, 502 P. 2d 1 (Cal: S. Ct. 1972). <scholar.google.com/scholar_case?case=9007336518867928085>.

186 Moore v. Regents of University of California, 793 P. 2d 479 (1990). <scholar.google.com/scholar_case?case=14543058709300681513>.

187 AMA Code of Medical Ethics, Opinion 2.1.1: Informed consent. <ama-assn.org/system/files/2019-06/code-of-medical-ethics-chapter-2.pdf>.

188 Cobbs v. Grant at 246, observing that patients may refuse to undergo a recommended treatment.

189 Shadrick v. Coker, 963 S.W. 2d 726, 732 (Tenn: Supreme Court 1998) ("the doctrine of lack of informed consent is based upon the tort of battery, not negligence").

Be Loyal, Honest, and Fair

Physicians also have a fiduciary duty to be completely loyal to the patient.[190] Physicians have an "ethical responsibility to place patients' welfare above the physician's own self-interest."[174] Physicians also must place the health of the patient ahead of obligations to others, such as to parents acting as legal proxies.

In addition, physicians have a fiduciary duty to be honest in all professional dealings.[191] Relatedly, they have a duty of good faith[192] and fair dealing.[193] Judge Benjamin Cardozo stated that fiduciaries are "held to something stricter than the morals of the marketplace. Not honesty alone, but the punctilio of an honor the most sensitive, is then the standard of behavior."[194] When people are in a fiduciary relationship, as here, any transaction between them must be "watched with extreme jealousy and solicitude; and if there is found the slightest trace of undue influence or unfair advantage, redress will be given to the injured party."[195]

Do Not Enrich Oneself At the Expense of One's Patient

Medicine is a caring profession, and most members of the profession are motivated by a desire to do what is best for each patient's health. For example, the admirable mission of the American Academy of Pediatrics is "to attain optimal physical, mental, and social health and well-being for all infants, children, adolescents and young adults."

<scholar.google.com/scholar_case?case=10687339754337651528>.

190 Pegram v. Herdrich, 530 U.S. 211, 235 (2000). The U.S. Supreme Court has observed that physicians have a fiduciary duty to act with "an eye single" toward the beneficiaries' interests. <scholar.google.com/scholar_case?case=17125855822711771249>.

191 AMA Code of Medical Ethics, Principle II. <ama-assn.org/sites/ama-assn.org/files/corp/media-browser/principles-of-medical-ethics.pdf>.

192 Lockett v. Goodill, 430 P.2d 589 (Wash. 1967). <scholar.google.com/scholar_case?case=7178094553151966468>.

193 Claims Arising from a Breach of Fiduciary Duty. NC Judges Handbook, at 18, citing cases. <ncbusinesslitigationreport.com/wp-content/uploads/sites/71/uploads/file/Judge%20Ervin%20Breach%20Fiduciary%20Duty.pdf>.

194 Meinhard v. Salmon, cited in Lawrence V. Cohn, 197 F. Supp. 2d 16 (SD NY D. Ct. 2002). <scholar.google.com/scholar_case?case=2567686355202108053>.

195 Cited in Eubanks v. Eubanks, 159 S.E. 2d 562 (1968); Fulp v. Fulp, 140 S.E.2d 708 (1965). <scholar.google.com/scholar_case?case=6147036455322326035>.

Of course, medicine is a profession as well. Like everyone else, physicians are naturally motivated by the desire and need to make money. Not surprisingly, however, physicians are not allowed to put their own financial interests ahead of the health and well-being of their patients. AMA Opinion 11.2.2 provides, "The primary objective of the medical profession is to render service to humanity; reward or financial gain is a subordinate consideration. Under no circumstances may physicians place their own financial interests above the welfare of their patients."[196]

That may be the rule, but the United States Supreme Court has recognized that physicians working for HMOs sometimes do provide unnecessary or useless services to improve the HMOs' profits,[190] which the HMO may give them a financial incentive to do.

Professors Hafemeister and Gulbrandsen explain that physicians have a fiduciary duty to deny requests for prescriptions that are medically contraindicated, even if it might alienate the patient and have adverse personal financial consequences for the physician.[197] In the context of circumcision, physicians have a financial interest in taking orders from parents to circumcise their son. If parents want their son circumcised, and a pediatrician performs the operation or approves it, he or she is also more likely to retain the child as a patient, and once again to make more money.

As discussed below, some physicians who circumcise are also motivated by a desire to preserve circumcision as a religious rite. Because physicians have a legal and ethical duty to provide competent medical care that patients' need, however, and to be completely loyal to the patient, physicians have a duty to suppress and disregard their own financial, religious, and other personal preferences in favor of the practice.

OBTAIN THE CONSENT OF A CHILD PATIENT WHENEVER POSSIBLE

What about minors? As a practical matter, physicians outside the United States virtually never operate on a healthy child. Healthy children do not

---

196 AMA Code of Medical Ethics, Opinion 11.2.2.<ama-assn.org/delivering-care/ethics/conflicts-interest-patient-care>.

197 Hafemeister TL, Gulbrandsen RM Jr. The Fiduciary Obligation of Physicians to Just Say No If an Informed Patient Demands Services that Are Not Medically Indicated. See note #164.

even meet the ordinary definition of a patient: "a sick individual especially when awaiting or under the care and treatment of a physician or surgeon."[198] Healthy children are not suitable candidates for surgery. Except for male genital cutting, physicians in the U.S. do not operate on healthy children either. Male genital cutting is therefore sui generis, from the Latin for "of its own kind." It is different or unique, unlike anything else in medicine or the law. It has been called "the elephant in the hospital."[199]

Circumcision is unlike anything else in medicine because it is not medicine. As Dr. Robert Van Howe attests in the attached affidavit, non-therapeutic circumcision falls outside the scope of the practice of medicine worldwide and in the United States.[200] In 2010, the Royal Dutch Medical Association similarly observed, "The rule is: do not operate on healthy children."[201] As discussed in Chapter 6 (Adults' and Children's Rights), that is indeed the rule.

The American Academy of Pediatrics' own Committee on Bioethics recognizes that children who have developed enough to be able to reason have the right to decide whether to undergo a medical procedure or not:

> Only patients who have appropriate decisional capacity and legal empowerment can give their *informed consent* to medical care. In all other situations, parents or other surrogates provide *informed permission* for diagnosis and treatment of children with the assent of the child whenever appropriate (emphasis added). ... Pediatric practice is unique in that developmental maturation allows, over time, for increasing inclusion of the child's and adolescent's opinion in medical decision-making in clinical practice and research. ... Health care providers should engage in the process of informed consent with [pediatric] patients before undertaking any medical intervention. ... [They]

---

198 Merriam-Webster Medical Dictionary, "patient."
  <merriam-webster.com/dictionary/patient#medicalDictionary>.
199 McAllister R. The Elephant in the Hospital. <youtu.be/lwevc3EELgl>.
200 Van Howe RS. Affidavit, Appendix, Para. 4.
201 Press release, Royal Dutch Medical Association (KNMG) to discourage non-therapeutic
  circumcision of male minors. 2010-05-27. <circinfo.org/Dutch_circumcision_policy.html>.

> should participate in decision-making commensurate with their
> development; they should provide assent to care whenever rea-
> sonable. … [The physician's] "[r]espect for competent patients'
> autonomy ordinarily extends even to the refusal or discontinua-
> tion [even] of their own life-sustaining treatment.[202]

The British Medical Association states to the same effect that it "cannot envisage a situation in which it is ethically acceptable to circumcise a competent, informed young person who consistently refuses the procedure." In fact, one refusal would be enough. But as discussed below, physicians in the United States sometimes *do* circumcise boys who make clear that they do not want to be circumcised, and thus over their objection. They also often badger parents to give permission even after the parents have refused the procedure.

Since every person in the United States has an absolute right to autonomy, circumcision must be deferred until a boy reaches the age of consent. There is no need to ask, and it is unfair to ask, older boys whether they want to be circumcised or not. Since medical professional do not tell parents the truth about the practice, they are unlikely to tell the boys the truth about it either. Moreover, the parents may pressure the boy to consent.

The only way for physicians and religious adherents to respect the rights of boys and men is to defer genital cutting until the legal age of consent when each boy can decide for himself (assuming that he ever thinks about it) whether he wants to be circumcised or not (invariably not).

CHAPTER SUMMARY

- Physicians must comply with the law and the rules of medical ethics and respect patients' rights.
- Physicians also have a fiduciary duty to act in the best interest of each patient. They must justify every medical procedure on medical

---

202 Roth-Cline M, Nelson RM, Parental Permission and Child Assent in Research on Children. *Yale J Biol Med.* 2013-09;86(3);291-301. <ncbi.nlm.nih.gov/pmc/articles/PMC3767214>

grounds; obtain the adult patient's fully informed consent whenever possible; be loyal, honest, and fair; and they are not allowed to enrich themselves at the expense of their patient.

- Physicians must also obtain the child's consent for an operation that the child needs whenever possible.
- The bottom line is that physicians are not allowed to operate on a healthy child. Physicians are required to defer any operation that can be deferred until a child reaches the age of consent. Hence, they are also not allowed to solicit parental permission for the operation.

8   PARENTS HAVE A DUTY TO PROTECT THEIR CHILD, AND THE RIGHT TO BE FULLY INFORMED

The legal scholar William Brigman discussed parents' rights and duties in the context of male circumcision in a 1985 article.[203] As he wrote, parents in the United States have custodial rights that give them wide latitude in how they raise their children, and courts are reluctant to become involved in family governance.[203] "The rights of parents to the care and custody of their children are not expressly set forth in the Constitution. However, the United States Supreme Court has upheld the fundamental rights of family integrity and recognized that there exists a private realm of family life beyond state control."[203] The Supreme Court has observed that parents have a fundamental "immediate right to the care, custody, management and companionship of minor children."[203] Courts thus give parents significant discretion or wide latitude in doing so.

PARENTS MUST RESPECT THEIR CHILD'S RIGHTS, AND THEY ARE NOT ALLOWED TO HARM THEIR CHILDREN

Nevertheless, parents do not own their children or their children's bodies, as the American circumcision industry would have the public and the parents of newborn boys believe. The U.S. physician Robert Van Howe writes that children have the full complement of human rights, and that parents do not have the right to completely control their children or to decide whether they will be circumcised or not. Rather, he claims, parents, "have an obligation to protect their children's rights as well as to preserve the future options of those children as far as possible." He concludes that the "notion that parents have a right to make decisions concerning their children's bodies and minds – irrespective of the child's best interests – is a dead dogma."[204]

The Supreme Court of California has confirmed this reasoning. "Children are not simply chattels belonging to the parent, but have funda-

203 Brigman WE. Circumcision as Child Abuse: The Legal and Constitutional Issues. *J Fam L.* 1985;23:337. <cirp.org/library/legal/brigman>.
204 Van Howe RS. Infant circumcision: the last stand for the dead dogma of parental (sovereignal) rights. *J Med Ethics.* 2013;7:475-81. <jme.bmj.com/content/39/7/475>.

mental interests of their own that may diverge from the interests of the parent."[136] Parents therefore, like physicians, must respect their child's rights under U.S. law and under international law, which is also part of U.S. law. As discussed in Chapter 6 (Adults' and Children's Rights), these includes the rights to bodily integrity, self-determination, privacy, freedom of religion, and equal protection of the law.

Courts often enter the family relationship to protect children. For example, parents can be held criminally liable for violating the child abuse statutes. As discussed in more detail in Chapter 22 (Fraudulent Legal Claims), parents cannot put their child's health and safety at risk or harm them for religious reasons either. As the legal scholar Karen Hughes writes, "neither the rights of religion nor the rights of parenthood are beyond limitation in matters affecting the child's welfare or when state action is necessary to protect the child against some clear and present danger."[205]

WHEN ACTING AS LEGAL REPRESENTATIVES OF THEIR SON, PARENTS HAVE DUTIES, NOT RIGHTS

When, unlike the case here, a child is suffering from a medical condition that must be treated, parents acting as legal proxies or as legal representatives of the child have legal duties to the child, not rights. After all, they are being called upon to make a medical decision as a representative of their child, on behalf of their child, as if standing in their child's shoes. When children need medical treatment and the treatment cannot be deferred, parents must try to determine what the child would have chosen; and if they are unable to do so, they must act in the child's best interests, without regard to their own personal preferences. AMA Code of Medical Ethics Opinion 2.1.2 makes this clear:

> Surrogate decision makers should base their decisions on the *substituted judgment standard;* in other words, they should use their knowledge of the patient's preferences and values to de-

---

205 Hughes K. The Criminalization of Female Genital Mutilation in the United States. See note #67; p. 351.

termine as best as possible what the patient would have decided herself. If there is not adequate evidence of the incapacitated or incompetent patient's preferences and values, the decision should be based on the *best interests of the patient* (what outcome would most likely promote the patient's well-being). Opinion 2.1.2 explains, 'Best interest decisions should be based on … the pain and suffering associated with the intervention,' 'the degree of and potential for benefit,' and 'impairments that may result from the intervention' (emphasis added).[206]

Applying the "substituted judgment" standard, parents must leave their children's genitals alone because, as discussed in Chapter 5 (Do Healthy People Want Their Genitals Cut Without Their Consent?), most boys would not choose to be circumcised if given the choice and able to make it. Even if one reached the "best interests" standard, the result would be the same. As several European courts have ruled (Chapter 12, European Cases), it is in the best interests of children not to expose them to the risks and harms of unnecessary genital surgery. Thus, parents are only allowed to elect to have their son circumcised in the rare case that it is medically necessary to do so – the last resort after all efforts to save the foreskin have failed.

The Bioethics Committee of the American Academy of Pediatrics considered the scope of parental authority in 1995 and reached the same conclusion that surrogates may only grant permission to treat a patient when the patient needs to be treated.

> Only patients who have appropriate decisional capacity and legal empowerment can give their informed consent to medical care. In all other situations, parents or other surrogates provide information permission for diagnosis and treatment of children with the assent of the child whenever appropriate.[207]

---

206 AMA Code of Medical Ethics Opinion 2.1.2. <ama-assn.org/system/files/2019-06/code-of-medical-ethics-chapter-2.pdf>

207 AAP Committee on Bioethics. Informed Consent, Parental Permission, and Assent in Pediatric Practice. *Pediatrics.* 1995-02;95(2):314-7. <pediatrics.aappublications.org/content/95/2/314>.

Furthermore, "In cases involving emancipated or mature minors with adequate decision-making capacity, or when otherwise permitted by law, physicians should seek informed consent directly from patients."[207] The committee also observed that "proxy consent" poses serious problems for pediatric health care providers. They "have legal and ethical duties to their child patients to render competent medical care based on what the patient needs, not what someone else expresses."[207] The Bioethics Committee of the British Medical Association expressed a similar view in 2019 in the context of circumcision. "Doctors are under no obligation to comply with a [parent's] request to circumcise a child."[208] In fact, they are under the obligation not to comply with a parent's request to do so.

Case law bears this out. The High Court of Australia, a common law jurisdiction like the United States, ruled in *Marion's Case* in 1992 that parents do not have the right to authorize the sterilization of a minor girl. Like sterilization, circumcision is non-therapeutic, excises normal, healthy functional tissue, is irreversible, and leaves the individual with permanently impaired physiological function. In the U.S. as well, according to a CNN article in 2007, "Report: 'Pillow angel' surgery broke law," a group vested with federal investigative authority for people with disabilities found that a hospital had violated a girl's constitutional and common law rights by performing a hysterectomy on her without a court order from the state. The hospital reportedly acknowledged its error and said that it was implementing changes to ensure that it will not sterilize another disabled child without a court order.

Similarly, the United States Supreme Court ruled in a 1979 case that parents do not have the right to institutionalize their child in a mental hospital. The court reasoned that "the child's rights and the nature of the commitment decision are such that parents do not always have absolute discretion to institutionalize a child." Parents might be mistaken in sincerely believing that their child needs to be institutionalized. Children should only be institutionalized when they need to be, as determined by a medical professional using independent medical judgment.[209] In short,

208 British Medical Association. The law and ethics of male circumcision: guidance for doctors. *J Med Ethics*. 2004;30(3). <jme.bmj.com/content/30/3/259>.
209 James Parham vs. J. R. et al., 442 U.S. 584 (1979). <law.cornell.edu/supremecourt/text/442/584>.

parents do not have the legal right to give permission to have their son institutionalized, or by analogy circumcised, except when a physician determines that it is medically necessary to do so.[210]

Thus, the longstanding claim by American medical associations, and more recently by the U.S. Centers for Disease Control and Prevention, that parents have the right to elect circumcision, and to take into consideration the parents' own religious, cultural, and personal aesthetic preferences in doing so, is simply false. In fact, the argument is knowingly false. Physicians are only licensed to practice medicine. They know that they are not allowed to take orders from parents to operate on a child for reasons having nothing to do with medicine. They know that what is in the best interests of the child may be different from what parents want. In fact, parents and religious adherents who give permission to circumcise healthy boys themselves commit criminal child abuse and a civil battery, just as medical professionals and religious practitioners do.

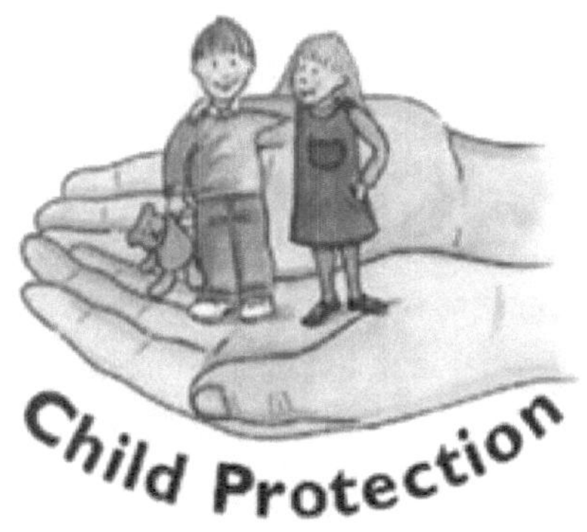

PARENTS HAVE THE RIGHT TO BE FULLY INFORMED WHEN MAKING MEDICAL DECISIONS

Although parents do not have the right to give permission for an operation on their healthy children, they have the right as legal proxies for their

---

210 Boyle GJ, Svobods JS, Price CP, Turner JN. Circumcision of Healthy Boys: Criminal Assault? *J L Med.* 2000-02;7:301-310. <cirp.org/library/legal/boyle1>.

children to approve or withhold approval for treatment that they need. In such a case the parents, like any patient, have the right to be fully informed about the recommended procedure, its hazards, and alternatives. Moreover, the physician has a duty to disclose to the decision maker(s) "all information relevant to a meaningful decision process."[211] Thus, unless parents are told literally *everything* that they might help them make an informed decision on behalf of their child, their permission is legally invalid, and they and their child have a legal claim against the physician and hospital for an unlawful battery.

Astonishingly, according to the Douglas Diekema, an ethicist at the American Academy of Pediatrics, half of the time medical professions do not give parents *any* information about circumcision.[212] Assuming that to be true, in at least half of all circumcisions performed in the United States, the circumcised boy, man, and his parents have a lawsuit against the physician and hospital for battery.

CHAPTER SUMMARY

- Parents do not own their child's body, and parents must respect their child's legal rights.
- When a child needs medical treatment, parents must choose what the child would have chosen, if given the choice and able to make it; and otherwise to choose what is in the best interests of the child's health.
- In making a medical decision on behalf of their child, parents are not allowed to take into consideration the parents' own religious, cultural, or other personal preferences.
- Parents who allow their son to be circumcised unwittingly commit criminal child abuse and a battery.

211 Cobbs v. Grant, 83 Cal. 3d 229, 235, 502 P.2d 1 (Cal. S. Ct. 1972).
<scholar.google.com/scholar_case?case=9007336518867928085>.
212 Diekema DS. Boldt v. Boldt: A pediatric ethics perspective. *J Clin Ethics*. 2009 Fall;20(3):251-7.
<pubmed.ncbi.nlm.nih.gov/19845198>.

Chapter 9 discusses how physicians bear the burden of justifying genital cutting. Chapter 10 discusses how circumcision is the perfect crime. Chapter 11 discusses the remedies available to boys, men, and their parents under U.S. civil law. Chapter 12 discusses European cases. Chapter 13 discusses American cases.

9   PHYSICIANS BEAR THE BURDEN OF JUSTIFYING GENITAL CUTTING

Ordinarily, a plaintiff in a civil case must prove the case by a preponderance of the evidence. "Under the preponderance standard, the burden of proof is met when the party with the burden convinces the fact finder (the jury) that there is a greater than 50% chance that the claim is true." The plaintiff needs to produce evidence showing that it is more likely that the claim is true than not. Consequently, the plaintiff ordinarily bears the "burden of proof" in a civil case.

During the first semester of law school, we learned that the outcome of litigation often depends upon which party bears the burden of proof. As an example, in O.J. Simpson's criminal trial, the state was unable to meet its burden of proving beyond a reasonable doubt that Simpson had murdered his wife – the legal standard for a criminal conviction. In the civil trial for "wrongful death," however, the plaintiffs were able to prove by a preponderance of the evidence or that it was more likely than not that he had killed his wife.[213] The reader might expect, therefore, that in a circumcision case in civil court, a circumcised boy or man would need to prove by a preponderance of the evidence that the physician acted unlawfully, but that is not the case.

Circumcision violates the plain wording of the child abuse statutes, and it satisfies the elements of, or what the plaintiff must prove to win a case of, battery and breach of fiduciary. In other words, it violates so-called "black letter" or well-established laws. Non-therapeutic genital cutting is therefore a so-called "prima facie" case of a child abuse, battery, and breach of fiduciary duty. "Prima facie" means on first encounter, at first sight,[214] or on its face. In legal terms, the allegation that a physician intruded into a person's body and cut off part of it creates a *rebuttable presumption* that the physician committed child abuse and acted unlawfully. The burden then falls to the physician to *rebut these presumptions*. To do so, the physician must assert a valid defense. Specifically, the

---

213 What's the difference between a civil judgment and a criminal conviction?" *NOLO.*
    <nolo.com/legal-encyclopedia/question-civil-judgment-versus-criminal-conviction-28300.html>.
214 "Prima facie." <en.wikipedia.org/wiki/Prima_facie>.

physician must provide a convincing medical reason why he or she is performing each procedure. Thirty-eight medical experts and ethicists representing pediatric medical associations in Northern Europe similarly noted in their critique of the AAP's 2012 circumcision guidelines that it is a generally accepted principle that physicians must justify all medical procedures performed on patients on medical grounds.[6] The British Medical Association likewise observed in its 2019 circumcision guidelines that physicians have a duty to justify circumcision. "As with any other aspect of care, health care professionals must be able to justify their decisions and should record the basis on which their decisions are made."[215]

In short, when a physician is about to operate on a patient (setting aside cosmetic surgery with adult consent), the physician must have a valid medical reason for doing so. As mentioned, the patient must be suffering from a medical condition requiring treatment; the physician must diagnose the medical condition; the physician must consider alternative treatment options, including the alternative of doing nothing; and the physician must determine and recommend the optimal treatment. Surgery is the optimal treatment and medically justified, however, only when it is medically necessary to treat the patient's medical condition. When the patient is a child, the operation also must be deferred until adulthood, whenever possible, to respect the patient's right to autonomy.[216] Thus, physicians are only allowed to operate on a child when the child needs an operation, and when it cannot be deferred until adulthood. It must be

---

215 British Medical Association. Non-therapeutic male circumcision (NTMC) of children – practical guidance for doctors. BMA circumcision policy statement. See #178, p. 15. <bma.org.uk/media/1847/bma-non-therapeutic-male-circumcision-of-children-guidance-2019.pdf>.
216 AMA Code of Medical Ethics, Opinion 8.08: Informed Consent. "The patient's right of self-decision can be effectively exercised only if the patient possesses enough information to enable an informed choice. The patient should make his or her own determination about treatment. The physician's obligation is to present the medical facts accurately to the patient or to the individual responsible for the patient's care and to make recommendations for management in accordance with good medical practice. The physician has an ethical obligation to help the patient make choices from among the therapeutic alternatives consistent with good medical practice. Informed consent is a basic policy in both ethics and law that physicians must honor, unless the patient is unconscious or otherwise incapable of consenting and harm from failure to treat is imminent." <journalofethics.ama-assn.org/article/ama-code-medical-ethics-opinions-informing-patients/2012-07>.

essential to the child's well-being to operate on him or her without delay, such as in a medical emergency or to prevent the child from dying.

Physicians in the U.S. who perform non-therapeutic circumcisions do not meet any of these requirements. Non-therapeutic means that the operation is not needed to treat a medical condition. Physicians do not weigh different options including the alternative of doing nothing, as required. The American Academy of Pediatrics has never recommended circumcision, and it stated in 2012 that it cannot recommend it. When my son was born, the physician did not recommend circumcision either. In fact, he told me that circumcision is not medically justified. When it comes to circumcision, then, physicians in the U.S. do not do what they are licensed to do, required to do, or do in every other case.

Rather, physicians tell the parents of newborn boys to weigh the medical pros and cons (which lay people are neither licensed nor able to do); and they let the parents decide whether the foreskin of their son's penis will be cut off or not. Thus, these physicians abdicate to parents their duty to use their independent medical judgment. The American Academy of Pediatrics even advises parents that they will need to weigh their own religious, cultural, and personal preferences in making the decision, which have nothing to do with medicine.

To summarize, the only way that a physician could rebut the presumption that every circumcision is unlawful is to prove that the child needed the operation, and that the operation could not be deferred until adulthood. Since healthy boys do not need the operation and it can be deferred until adulthood, physicians will never be able to meet their burden of justifying the operation. Of course, physicians will continue to attempt to justify the practice, as they have been doing for the past 150 years, but they will never be able to do so. This explains why whenever one reason is refuted, physicians need to propose a new one, mostly recently, "prevents HIV!"

CHAPTER SUMMARY

- Every person has a right to bodily integrity, self-determination, and privacy.

- An operation violates those rights and is a prima facie or rebuttable case of an unlawful battery.
- To rebut that presumption, physicians bear the burden of proving that the operation was medically necessary and that it could not be deferred until adulthood.
- Because it is not necessary to cut a boy's penis and the operation can be deferred until adulthood, it will never be possible for physicians to justify the practice.

10   THE PERFECT CRIME

This chapter shows that it is a crime for a physician to circumcise a healthy boy, and that the implications are profound.

CRIMINAL CHILD ABUSE

Any person who cuts off any part of a girl's genitals, including the prepuce or clitoral hood, violates the plain wording of the child abuse statutes in every state.[217] For example, New York State defines "abused child" as occurring when a parent or other person legally responsible for a child's care, thus including a physician, "inflicts or allows to be inflicted upon the child physical injury ... which causes or creates a substantial risk of death, serious or protracted disfigurement, protracted impairment of physical or emotional health or protracted loss or impairment of the function of any bodily organ." A sex offense against a child also constitutes child abuse. In order to defend against a charge of child abuse, the physician would need to prove that it was medically necessary to cut off part of the girl's genitals. Notably, physicians are also required to report suspected cases of child abuse for investigation and prosecution when child abuse has occurred.[218,219]

In 2015, a senior British judge reasoned that since any form of female genital mutilation constitutes "significant harm" under the United Kingdom Children Act of 1989, and since some forms of female genital mutilation are less invasive than male circumcision, the latter constitutes

---

217 Silver S, Green R. A Guide to New York's Child Protective Services System. 2001:9. (defining "abused child" in New York as when a parent or other person legally responsible for a child's care, such as a physician, "inflicts or allows to be inflicted upon the child physical injury ... which causes or creates a substantial risk of death, serious or protracted disfigurement, protracted impairment of physical or emotional health or protracted loss or impairment of the function of any bodily organ," and it prohibits a sex offense against the child.)

218 Id. at 11.

219 See also: Black L. Liability for Failure to Report Child Abuse. *AMA J Ethics.* 2007-12. ("When a physician is faced with possible cases of child abuse, that physician must report the injuries to the proper authorities.") <journalofethics.ama-assn.org/article/liability-failure-report-child-abuse/2007-12>.

a "significant harm" as well.[220] When harm is significant, the penalty is a longer prison term.[221]

In 1985, the legal scholar William Brigman observed that children have been abused in wide variety of ways since the beginning of recorded history. (One example is foot binding, the custom in Imperial China of breaking and tightly binding the feet of young girls as a mark of feminine beauty. Foot binding is analogous to circumcision, which parents often elect because they prefer the appearance of the circumcised penis.) Brigman showed that male genital cutting, like female genital cutting, violates the criminal child abuse statutes in every U.S. state. He reasoned,

> [C]hild abuse, commonly defined as the intentional, non-accidental use of physical force that results in injury to a child, is universally proscribed by state law. The California law is typical: '[C]hild abuse' means a physical injury which is inflicted by other than accidental means on a child by another person. … Since [male] circumcision is not medically warranted, has no significant physiological benefits, is painful because it is performed without anesthesia and leaves a wound in which urinary salts burn, carries a significant risk of surgical complications, including death, and deforms the penis, it would seem that as a nonaccidental physical injury, it is properly included in the definition of child abuse.[203]

Circumcision meets the definition of physical injury under Massachusetts child abuse law, which includes impairment of any organ and any non-trivial injury. Moreover, because male genital cutting permanently disfigures the penis compared to its intact state, disables the mobile functions of the foreskin vis-à-vis the rest of the penis, and carries many minor and serious medical risks including death, it meets the definition of a substantial harm in some states, as defined in some state child abuse

---

220 Re B and G (Children) [2015] EWFC 3 LJ13C00295, [9, 22]. <familylaw.co.uk/news_and_comment/re-b-and-g-children-no-2-2015-ewfc-3>.

221 MASS. GEN. LAWS c. 265, § 13J(a)–(b) (establishing a prison term of "not more than fifteen years" for assault causing "substantial bodily injury" to a child, compared to five years for more minor assaults).

statutes.[222,223] In 2010, in $\boxed{\textit{Williamson v. State of Texas}}$ – a Texas appeals court case involving unnecessary surgery on a child that caused serious bodily injury – a physician testified that "unnecessary surgeries do not constitute reasonable medical care."[224] The court held that the physician's use of a scalpel constituted use of a deadly weapon in violation of a Texas criminal child abuse statute.[225]

It is also noteworthy that a few states (Illinois, Idaho, and formerly California) have statutes that exempt circumcision from ritual abuse statutes. The only reason that legislators would enact such legislation is that circumcision *is* ritual abuse and child abuse,[226] but physicians do not want to be prosecuted for it. Since circumcision is unconstitutional and a crime, those statutes are invalid.

As discussed in Chapter 22 (Fraudulent Legal Claims), parents cannot defend against a charge of child abuse by claiming that they were motivated by a sincerely held religious belief. The only valid defense or excuse that a physician or a parent could assert is that the child needed the operation. In short, "[t]here is no reason, other than cultural bias, why the current child abuse laws and laws prohibiting female circumcision are not applied to those performing involuntary male circumcision."[227]

CRIMINAL ASSAULT

In 1997, the Canadian ethicist Margaret A. Somerville, "characterized male circumcision as 'technically criminal assault' under the Canadian

---

222 Definitions of Child Abuse and Neglect. Child Welfare Information Gateway.

223 See also M.G.L. c. 265, § 13L ("Whoever wantonly or recklessly engages in conduct that creates a substantial risk of serious bodily injury or sexual abuse to a child or wantonly or recklessly fails to take reasonable steps to alleviate such risk where there is a duty to act shall be punished by imprisonment in the house of correction for not more than 21/2 years."
"'Serious bodily injury" [is] bodily injury which results in a permanent disfigurement, protracted loss or impairment of a bodily function, limb or organ, or substantial risk of death").

224 Williamson v. State, 356 S.W. 3d 1, 15 (Ct. App. Tx. 2010). <scholar.google.com/scholar_case?case=10994570214431513519>.

225 Id. at 27.

226 See, e.g., the Illinois ritual sexual abuse statute (2015).
See the discussion of the Idaho ritual abuse law here: <religioustolerance.org/ra_law.htm>.
The exemption is at b(2). California's 1995 ritual abuse law exemption circumcision was section 667.83 of the California Penal Code, Section 3), but the law was repealed in 1997.

227 Van Howe RS, et al. Involuntary Circumcision: The Legal Issues. *BJU Int.* 1999;83:63,73.

criminal code."[228] In 1997, Christopher Price,[229] an Oxford trained international and human rights lawyer, reasoned similarly that because it is non-therapeutic, invasive, and irreversible, surgery with serious potential risks, it violates the common law assault provisions of Queensland, Australia's Criminal Code.[230] He observed that this has been clearly established in the case of female genital cutting, including minor forms that are less invasive than penile circumcision.[229] Canada and Australia are both common law jurisdictions like the United States.

Likewise, in a landmark decision in 2012, a regional court in Cologne, Germany held that circumcision is unlawful,[231] for the first time since the Romans had made it a capital crime in ancient times. Moreover, the German court ruled that it is an assault and a crime for a physician to circumcise a boy for religious reasons, and by implication, whenever it is performed without medical need.[232] The court found that the practice causes an irreversible and harmful injury. It found that non-therapeutic circumcision violates Article 2 of the German constitution, which stipulates: "Every person shall have the right to life and physical integrity." (That is also a rule of European law applicable to all European countries.) The court reasoned that a boy's right to bodily integrity and self-determination supersedes his parents' religious and other rights.[232,233] Consequently, parents cannot provide valid consent for the procedure.[232] It must be delayed until an age at which the boy can choose for himself whether to have it performed.

Under political pressure from Israel, and over the objection of the German Pediatric Association and other European medical associations,

---

228 Circumcision: Legal issues. *Circumcision Information and Resource Pages.*
   <cirp.org/library/legal/>
229 Price C. Male Circumcision: An Ethical and Legal Affront. *Bull Med Ethics.* 1997-05;128:13-9.
   <cirp.org/library/legal/price>.
230 Circumcision of Male Infants Research Paper, *Queensland L Reform Comm'n.* Brisbane
   (1993).
231 Kulish N. German Ruling Against Circumcising Boys Draws Criticism. *NY Times.* 2012-06-26.
   <nytimes.com/2012/06/27/world/europe/german-court-rules-against-circumcising-boys.html>.
232 Landgericht Köln [Cologne Regional Court] May 7, 2012, Urteil Ns 169/11 (Germany). English
   translation provided by Professor Holm Putzke available from the author.
233 Wendy Zeldin, Germany: Regional Court Ruling Criminalizes Circumcision of Young Boys.
   Library of Congress: Global Legal Monitor. 2012-07-03.
   <loc.gov/law/foreign-news/article/germany-regional-court-ruling-criminalizes-circumcision-of-young-boys>.

the German legislature subsequently passed a specific statute allowing religious circumcisions.[141] The legislation was thus politically motivated and enacted despite the warnings of Germany's medical profession. Reinhard Merkel and Holm Putzke suggest that the German government felt compelled to allow Jews to continue their rite of circumcision due to guilt about the genocidal mass murder of Jews in Germany during the Nazi era. They reason, however, that if circumcision were not an ancient and sacred religious ritual of Jews, and if Jews proposed it as a new ritual today, the law would not tolerate it. In other words, societies give circumcision a pass because it is a longstanding religious and cultural practice, even though it is bad for the health of boys and men. Importantly, Merkel and Putzke conclude that circumcision remains unlawful notwithstanding the special statute, as it still meets the definition of assault under German law.[141]

MANSLAUGHTER

As discussed above, 1 in 50,000 circumcisions results in a fatality. Approximately 1.5 million boys are circumcised per year in the U.S. resulting in about thirty deaths per year. (Moreover, since about one-third of all boys worldwide are circumcised, often in unsterile settings, the number of deaths worldwide each year must be large.) Those deaths are all avoidable and constitute manslaughter under U.S. law, homicide that is the unintentional killing of another person.

THE PERFECT CRIME

The perfect crime has been defined as "a crime so ingeniously contrived and carefully executed that it cannot be detected or solved." Physicians who perform circumcisions and their hospitals have been committing criminal child abuse, criminal assault, and occasionally manslaughter on boys in the United States for the past 150 years, and they get away with it. How can that be?

One reason is that boys and men may not even be aware that they have been circumcised. If they were circumcised at birth, they will not remember the pain. They may believe the American medical profession's false portrayal of circumcision as good for health on the one hand and as the harmless snip of a useless piece of skin on the other. They are unlikely to know that doctors deprived them of the most sensitive part of their penis.[120] And until the German court ruling that circumcision is criminal assault became front page news, the practice was rarely discussed in public in the United States.

State governments call upon people who know of or suspect child abuse to report it to the authorities, the police, and state attorneys general. When they do, however, the authorities do not know that it is crime, so they do not prosecute the physicians.[234] They perceive it to be medicine. So long as physicians and their medical/trade associations defend the practice, it is very difficult to persuade the authorities that it is harmful, let alone that it is also unlawful and child abuse.

Whether performed by physicians or religious adherents, unnecessary genital cutting is therefore the perfect crime. It is also the perfect fraud, so well hidden from the public, people who know little or nothing about medicine or law, that it has endured for 150 years.

IMPLICATIONS

One implication of the fact that non-therapeutic genital cutting is a crime is that every time a physician circumcises a boy in the United States, the physician risks being prosecuted, jailed for several years, and fined. One day a physician in Germany was circumcising a boy for religious reasons, and shortly thereafter a regional court determined that in doing so he was committing a crime.

Secondly, statutes that authorize doing anything illegal are void, as are contracts. Therefore, the legislation in some states attempting to exempt circumcision from state ritual abuse statutes are void. Federal or state legislation allowing circumcision would be void.

In addition, as the United States Supreme Court observed in 1899, "The authorities from the earliest time [in England] to the present unanimously hold that no court will lend its assistance in any way towards

____

234 Video of an unsuccessful effort to report circumcision as child abuse: <youtu.be/T8I-V59Tn00>.

carrying out the terms of an illegal contract." It is an absolute defense to the enforcement of any contract that it involves engaging in an illegal activity. Therefore, every contract involving circumcision is legally invalid, unenforceable, and void. These contracts include advertisements for circumcision; marketing materials; the parents' verbal election of circumcision; the consent forms that parents sign; the billing codes that physician use for circumcision; private insurance contracts authorizing payments for it; Medicaid agreements to pay for circumcision; invoices by physicians and hospitals for reimbursement; and contracts for the sale and resale of the unlawfully harvested foreskins.

CHAPTER SUMMARY

- It is criminal child abuse for a physician, a nurse, a religious practitioner, or a lay person to circumcise a healthy boy or girl, and for a parent to give permission for it.
- Non-therapeutic circumcision is also criminal assault. When the child dies, the physician has committed involuntary manslaughter.
- Circumcision is the perfect crime. The police do not know that it is a crime. It is the perfect fraud as well. Circumcised males, their parents, and the public do not know that they have been deceived.
- Every time a physician circumcises a boy, he or she risks being jailed for several years and fined.
- Exemptions for ritual abuse and any future legislation allowing unnecessary genital cutting are void.
- Because male genital cutting is a crime, every statute and every contract involving it is void.

11   Remedies Under U.S. Civil Law

At a debate about whether circumcision is legal or not, the only argument that the physician Michael Brady of the American Academy of Pediatrics 2012 committee on circumcision could muster in favor of its legality was that no physician in the United States has ever been held liable for properly performing the procedure.[235] Dr. Brady's claim is true, but it does not follow that circumcision is lawful. For example, slavery was once common in the United States, but it was not only a moral abomination but an unconstitutional violation of natural rights before the Thirteenth Amendment abolished it.[236] Similarly, no court in Germany had ruled that circumcision is criminal assault under German law either until 2012, but it was a crime before that nonetheless: the law simply had not been prosecuted. Given that circumcision violates boys' and men's rights, what remedies do boys and men who have been circumcised and their parents have in U.S. courts, applying general principles of law? What "causes of action" or claims can they bring in lawsuits?

Adults' Claims Arising From Unnecessary Non-Consensual Surgery

A shocking amount of unnecessary surgery is performed on adults in the United States.[236] In a 2017 article, three surgeons attributed this to the profitable nature of the practice and the reluctance of surgeons to abandon procedures that they have learned, even when strong evidence shows that they have no medical benefit.[236] There are two types of unnecessary surgery: surgery on healthy people – who of course do not need an operation – and surgery on patients who are suffering from a medical condition that is not in their best interests because more conservative treatment

---

235 Debate between J. Steven Svoboda, Executive Director of Attorneys for the Right of the Child, and Michael Brady & Douglas Diekema, Task Force on Circumcision, American Academy of Pediatrics, at The Twentieth Pitts Lectureship in Medical Ethics at the University of South Carolina in Charleston, South Carolina. 2013-10-18/19. <arclaw.org/debates/arc-releases-video-from-charleston-debate-victory-over-american-academy-of-pediatrics>.

236 Barnett RE. Was Slavery Unconstitutional Before the Thirteenth Amendment? Lysander Spooner's Theory of Interpretation. *Pac L J*. 1997;28:977-1013. <scholarship.law.georgetown.edu/facpub/1238>.

alternatives exist, or because it would be better to do nothing. The book focuses on the former, where there is no question that the surgery is unnecessary.

The three surgeons observed that medical malpractice suits have not stemmed from the practice. Even seasoned trial lawyers might believe that unnecessary non-consensual surgery gives rise to a medical malpractice lawsuit.[236] The prefix "mal" in malpractice, however, means "bad," from the Latin word *malus*. Thus, malpractice claims involve surgery that has been performed badly, negligently, or below the accepted standard of proper medical care expected of physicians. "The relevant issue in a medical malpractice action is whether the diagnosis or treatment violated the applicable standard of care and thereby caused the plaintiff's injury."[237] A possible defense to a malpractice action is that other surgeons or physicians also perform the same surgery the same way, so the treatment met the standard of care in a community. Physicians are liable for performing unnecessary surgery on a healthy person without consent, by contrast, not because they made a mistake in diagnosing the patient's medical condition, or performed the operation badly or negligently, but rather because the person did not need any treatment. In short, liability for unnecessary surgery arises because the physician should not have performed the operation at all.[238]

As mentioned above, in *Tortorella v. Castro,*[167] a California appeals court held that unnecessary surgery on a healthy adult without fully informed consent as in the case of elective cosmetic surgery is unlawful, but the court did not specify what causes of action or claims the plaintiff could bring in a lawsuit. The case of *Lloyd v. Kramer*[239] is instructive in that regard. There, a physician told a woman suffering from a medical condition that she needed abdominal surgery, when her medical condition could have been treated without surgery. The court allowed the plaintiff

---

237 King v. Sowers, 471 S.E.2d 481 (Va: S. Ct. 1996). <scholar.google.com/scholar_case?case=7448978490769130095>.

238 See the dissenting opinion in Demers v. Gerety, 529 P.2d 278, 282 (NM: Ct. App. 1974). "The majority opinion limits its discussion of negligent surgery ... that defendant failed to perform the operation with care and skill. This is incorrect because defendant should not have performed the operation at all." <scholar.google.com/scholar_case?case=4346552828424490190>.

239 Lloyd v. Kramer, 503 S.E. 2d 632 (Ga: Ct. App. 1998). <scholar.google.com/scholar_case?case=9706643766065218208>.

to proceed to trial on her claims for *battery* (an unlawful touching), for *breach of fiduciary duty* (a breach of trust), and for *fraud* (intentionally fraudulent representation), as the physician had falsely claimed that she needed surgery when she did not.

CHILDREN'S CLAIMS ARISING FROM GENITAL CUTTING

What about minors subjected to medically unnecessary genital cutting? Children have the same legal rights as adults. They are also entitled to the additional protection of the child abuse statutes by reason of their minority and vulnerability. The genitals are given even more protection by law from non-consensual interference, whether by touching or cutting, by the states that have extended the statute of limitations (the length of time during which claims can be made) for sexual abuse.

Female Genital Cutting Is Analogous

For example, in 1996, the United States Congress passed legislation, a federal statute, holding that female genital cutting is a crime, except when it is medically necessary. Congress made findings and reasoned:

> The Congress finds that – (1) the practice of female genital mutilation is carried out by members of certain cultural and religious groups within the United States; (2) the practice of female genital mutilation often results in the occurrence of physical and psychological health effects that harm the women involved; (3) *such mutilation infringes upon the guarantees of rights secured by Federal and State law, both statutory and constitutional* ... (emphasis added).[240]

Parenthetically, in 2018 a U.S. District Court judge ruled that this federal statute is unconstitutional.[241] He reasoned that female genital mutilation

---

240 Omnibus Consolidated Appropriations Act of 1997, Pub. L. No. 104-208, § 645, 709-10.
241 Earp BD. Why Was the U.S. Ban on Female Genital Mutilation Ruled Unconstitutional, and What Does This Have to Do with Male Circumcision? *Ethics Med & Pub Health.* 2022-07. <researchgate.net/publication/341965054>.

is a criminal activity that only states can regulate and not the federal government. Whether that ruling stands or not, the reasoning of the U.S. Congress in passing the legislation was correct. Female genital cutting is harmful and violates girls' rights; their rights supersede their parents' rights, including their parents' religious rights; and girls subjected to genital cutting have legal remedies. This accords with the European and UK cases that have ruled that the child's right to be free from genital cutting supersedes the parents' religious and other rights. Non-therapeutic male and female genital cutting give rise to the following legal claims in civil lawsuits.

Civil Battery

Svoboda, Van Howe, and Dwyer wrote in 2000, "The common law has always recognized battery – violation of a person's right to be free from unwanted touching – as a civil and criminal wrong."[242] The elements of the civil claim of battery are: "(1) defendant intentionally performed an act that resulted in a harmful or offensive contact with the plaintiff's person; (2) plaintiff did not consent to the contact; and (3) the harmful or offensive contact caused injury, damage, loss or harm to plaintiff."[243] Cutting off part of a person's penis certainly meets that definition. As discussed, the court in *Lloyd v. Kramer,* involving unnecessary foot surgery on an adult, allowed the plaintiff's battery claim to proceed to trial.[239]

Unnecessary non-consensual genital surgery constitutes a rebuttable case of assault under the criminal law and a rebuttable case of battery under the civil law. (Cosmetic surgery on an adult also constitutes an assault and battery, but the violence is justified by the fully informed consent of the person being subjected to it. In such a case, physicians can rebut the presumption that the invasion of the body is an assault and battery.)

---

242 Svoboda JS, et al. Informed Consent for Neonatal Circumcision: An Ethical and Legal Conundrum. *J Contemp Health L & Policy.* 2000;17:61.

243 Brown v. Ransweiler, 171 Cal. App. 4th 516, 526-27 (Cal: Court of Appeal, 4th App. Dist., 1st Div. 2009). <scholar.google.com/scholar_case?case=11432781847804866510>.

As discussed above, the same reasoning applies in the United States to male and female genital cutting. The only exception that Congress carved out for female genital cutting is that it is lawful when it is medically necessary.[244] Likewise, male genital cutting is lawful only when it is medically necessary and cannot be deferred. Thus, it is a battery – both a civil tort (a wrong giving rise to a claim in civil court) and a crime (subject to prosecution, jail time, and a fine) – for a physician to circumcise a healthy boy.

The court in Cologne, Germany in 2012 ruled that not only the physician, but also his parents, had committed the crime of assault in choosing to have their son circumcised for religious reasons. Parents in the U.S. who elect to have their son circumcised likewise, though unwittingly, violate the child abuse statutes, commit criminal assault against their child, and a civil battery, as do religious practitioners who perform the most circumcisions worldwide.

Accordingly, circumcised boys and men have the right to sue the physician, hospital, or the religious practitioner, and technically even their parents, for battery. Nothing would be gained from it, though, as the parents could sue the physician and hospital, and that would irrevocably harm the parent-child relationship. Upon winning, the boys and men would have a right to compensatory damages, including for pain and suffering during and after the operation, for loss of the foreskin, and for any resulting psychological harm.

False Imprisonment

Physicians are required to discharge children they pronounce healthy from the hospital at the earliest opportunity. Healthy children are not suitable candidates for surgery. Since it is illegal and indeed a crime to operate on a healthy child, this also gives rise to a claim for the tort of false imprisonment. The Restatement 2d on Torts § 35: False Imprisonment provides:

---

244 Legislation on Female Genital Mutilation in the United States, Center For Reproductive Rights. 2004; at 3.

(1) An actor is liable for false imprisonment if: (a) he acts intending to confine the other or a third person within boundaries fixed by the actor, and (b) his act directly or indirectly results in such a confinement of the other, and (c) the other is conscious of the confinement or is harmed by it.[245]

Breach of Fiduciary Duty

As discussed in Chapter 7 (Physicians' Duties), physicians have a fiduciary duty, or a duty based on trust, to act in the best interests of each patient, keeping the best interests of the patient paramount. As discussed in Chapter 12 (European Cases), it is in the best interests of healthy boys not to circumcise them.

The Queensland Law Reform Commission in Australia, a common law country like the United States, concluded that it is in a boy's best interest to respect his bodily integrity[246] and not to circumcise him unless it is medically necessary.[247] The court in Cologne, Germany and a court in the United Kingdom, another common law country, both held that it is in the best interests of two boys to respect their right to autonomy and defer circumcision until the boys reached adulthood.[248] The United States Supreme Court is in accord with this reasoning as it stated in *Pegram v. Herdrich* that "excessive surgery is not in the patient's best interest."[190] Excessive surgery is more surgery than a person needs and it therefore encompasses surgery that a person does not need.

There is a specific ethical rule prohibiting physicians from performing unnecessary surgery.[249] Non-therapeutic circumcision also violates the

---

245 The Restatement 2d on Torts § 35: False Imprisonment.
246 Stilwell v. Walden, 320 S.E. 2d 329, 332 (NC 1984) ("It is just because confidence in others inherently and inevitably begets influence that the law of constructive fraud is needed, lest that influence be exerted for the benefit of the one having it, rather than that of the one whose confidence created it.") <scholar.google.com/scholar_case?case=6075830575755308449>.
247 Queensland Law Reform Commission.
248 Re L and B (Children) (Specific Issues: Temporary Leave to Remove from the Jurisdiction; Circumcision), [2016] EWHC 849 (Fam) FD12P01761, 143 (Eng.).
249 AMA Opinion 11.2.2, "Conflicts of Interest in Patient Care," provides: "The primary objective of the medical profession is to render service to humanity; reward or financial gain is a subordinate consideration. Under no circumstances may physicians place their own financial interests above the welfare of their patients. [Para.] Treatment or hospitalization that is willfully exces-

fundamental rules of medical ethics. These include: autonomy; non-male-ficence (do no harm); the rule of proportionality (do more good than do harm, and do the least amount of harm); and the rule of justice, because it is unfair to circumcise a boy who would not have chosen it for himself and who is powerless to prevent it.[250] The ethical violations also constitute breaches of the fiduciary duty that physicians owe to each patient.

In addition, as quoted above, "physicians breach their fiduciary duty to patients when they abdicate their responsibility to exercise independent medical judgment and provide their patients with access to medical services that are not medically indicated."[251] Unnecessary genital cutting violates the physician's fiduciary duty of loyalty: it puts the physician's own self-interests ahead of what is in the best interests of boys and men; and it puts the demands of parents ahead of what is best for the overall health of boys and men. In addition, as shown in Part IV, physicians do not tell parents – who are representing their son on his behalf – the truth about circumcision, which violates physicians' duty to be honest and constitutes intentional fraud.

Unjust Enrichment

Like breach of fiduciary duty, unjust enrichment is a claim arising from a physician's breach of trust. Male genital cutting unjustly enriches physicians at the expense of their patients. As shown in Chapter 15 (Undisclosed Conflicts of Interest and Motives to Defraud), circumcision is a multibillion dollar per year industry.

sive or inadequate constitutes unethical practice. Physicians should not provide wasteful and unnecessary treatment that may cause needless expense solely for the physician's financial benefit or for the benefit of a hospital or other health care organization with which the physician is affiliated. [Para.] Where the economic interests of the hospital, health care organization, or other entity are in conflict with patient welfare, patient welfare takes priority. [Para.] This opinion underscores that, above all, *the interests of a patient and beneficence must take precedence over a physician's or institution's financial gain* (emphasis added)." <journalofethics.ama-assn.org/article/ama-code-medical-ethics-opinions-related-organizational-influence-health-care/2020-03>.

250 Doctors Opposing Circumcision. Medical Ethics and the Non-Therapeutic Circumcision of Male Children. 2016-06. <doctorsopposingcircumcision.org/for-professionals/medical-ethics>.

251 Hafemeister TL, Gulbrandsen RM Jr. The Fiduciary Obligation of Physicians to Just Say No If an Informed Patient Demands Services that Are Not Medically Indicated. See note #164, p. 376.

Violation of Consumer Protection Statutes

Finally, many states have enacted consumer protection statutes to protect consumers who may lack knowledge, experience, or capacity from any false, misleading, unfair, deceptive, bad faith, or unconscionable trade practice.[252] In North Carolina, conduct that constitutes a breach of fiduciary duty and constructive fraud is sufficient to support an unfair and deceptive trade practice claim.[253,254] Insofar as physicians use unfair and deceptive practices to sell circumcision, even though it is unlawful and a crime, it may well violate a state's consumer protection act, depending upon the statute's wording.

CHAPTER SUMMARY

- Unnecessary surgery without consent is unlawful.
- Adults subjected to unnecessary surgery without their consent have claims for battery (an unlawful touching); false imprisonment; breach of fiduciary duty (breach of trust); unjust enrichment (enriching the physician at the expense of the patient); and violation of many state consumer protection statutes (unfair and deceptive practices).
- Children subjected to unnecessary genital cutting have these same civil claims as adults.

252 Mass. Gen. Laws, ch. 93A, § 2 (2020).
<malegislature.gov/Laws/GeneralLaws/Parti/Titlexv/Chapter93a/Section2>.
253 Darviris v. Petros, 442 Mass. 274, 279 (2004) (listing cases holding that unfair trade practice suits against doctors are limited to business activities, such as billing and advertising, and not medical activities). <scholar.google.com/scholar_case?case=11544464367090750859>.
254 N.C. Judges Handbook, Breach of Fiduciary Duty Claims, citing cases.
<ncbusinesslitigationreport.com/wp-content/uploads/sites/71/uploads/file/Judge%20Ervin%20Breach%20Fiduciary%20Duty.pdf>

12 EUROPEAN CASES

This chapter discusses how European medical associations have called circumcision medically indefensible; how several European governments have considered banning it; and how a consensus has emerged in court cases in Europe, including the United Kingdom, that the practice is harmful and unlawful. (Most of this chapter has been taken from an article, *"Circumcision is Unethical and Unlawful,"* that Steven Svoboda, Robert Van Howe, and I published in the *Journal of Law and Medical Ethics* in 2016. Where citations are not provided, they are in the original.)

MEDICAL ASSOCIATIONS

Medical associations in Western countries other than the U.S. agree that there is no medical basis for circumcision, and they are calling for the regulation, restriction, and even prohibition of circumcision to defend boys' rights to physical integrity. In 2012, the German Federal Association of Pediatricians (BVKJ) opposed the bill that later became law in Germany, and supported alternative legislation that would have respected boys' right to bodily integrity. It also strongly criticized the American Academy of Pediatrics' 2012 circumcision policy statement and technical report. On September 28, 2013, Sweden's Ombudsman for Children, and representatives of four leading Swedish physicians' organizations, stated, "To circumcise a child without medical reasons and without the child's consent, runs contrary ... to the child's human rights and the fundamental principles of medical ethics." The Royal Dutch Medical Association and the South African Medical Association also have concluded that male circumcision constitutes a human rights violation and should be legally restricted in most cases or at the very least strictly regulated. The Swedish Medical Association, which includes 85% of the country's doctors, recommends setting a minimum age for the procedure and requiring the boy's consent. The Danish College of General Practitioners issued a statement that ritual circumcision of boys is tantamount to abuse and mutilation. The Finnish Medical Association has stated, "child circumcisions are in conflict with medical ethics." The Swedish Pediatric Society has called infant male circumcision an "assault on boys."

LEGISLATIVE BODIES

A similar consensus is emerging among legislators, courts, and similar bodies in developed countries outside the United States that circumcision violates the rights of the child. The Tasmania Law Reform Institute recommended strict regulation of the practice, and legal prohibition in most cases, with limited exemptions for religious and cultural observance. On July 4, 2013, the United Nations' Committee on the Rights of the Child, which oversees nation states' compliance with the Convention on the Rights of the Child, issued a document in which it "expressed concern about reported short and long-term complications arising from some traditional male circumcision practices." On September 24, 2013, Swedish legislators introduced a bill that would have outlawed the circumcision of males younger than 18 years of age for non-medical reasons. On October 1, 2013, the Council of Europe passed a recommendation endorsing a child's right to physical integrity, as well as a resolution supporting genital autonomy for children by opposing several practices including male circumcision, female genital cutting, and "early childhood medical interventions in the case of intersexual children." A draft law in Finland in 2014 aimed at banning circumcision received substantial support from Finnish legislators, the majority of whom supported either banning or limiting it. Iceland and Denmark also considered legislation banning circumcision. The bills did not pass, but likely only out of deference to religious advocates of the practice.

COURTS

Several European cases have upheld a boy's right to bodily integrity, as reported by Attorneys for the Rights of the Child, which translated the decisions that were not written in English.[255]

---

255 <arclaw.org/projects/arc-publishes-trove-of-translated-european-legal-documents>.

In a July 2007 case in Austria, a child's biological mother sought the procedure for hygienic reasons over the opposition of both foster parents. The court ruled that circumcision is unlawful, reasoning that it is irreversible, not medically necessary, and not in the best interests of the child. In a 2007 case in the Netherlands, the court ruled that circumcision is not in the child's best interests. In a September 2007 case, a German appeals court found that the circumcision by a physician of an 11-year-old boy, without his approval, constituted an unlawful personal injury. As discussed, in a landmark decision in 2012, a regional court in Cologne, Germany ruled that circumcision for religious reasons is harmful and criminal assault. In 2013, another German court held that a German born woman of Kenyan descent could not authorize doctors to circumcise a six-year-old child of whom she had custody because it might cause him psychological harm. Also in 2013, a Swiss court prohibited a parent from circumcising her son "under the threat of punishment formulated in Art. 292 of the Swiss Criminal Code."[256]

Proponents of the practice might argue that Germany, the Netherlands, Austria, and Switzerland are civil law countries, whereas the United States is a common law country. General principles of law appear to be largely the same, however, under either body of law. For example, it is European Union law that member countries must respect a person's right to personal security or bodily integrity. In any event, two courts in the United Kingdom, a common law country like the United States, have issued similar opinions.

In January 2015, in a case involving female genital cutting, a UK judge stated, "In my judgment, if FGM Type IV [the least harmful form of FGC] amounts to significant harm, as in my judgment it does, then the same must be so of male circumcision." The Yale ethics Brian Earp commented, "The importance of this conclusion cannot be overstated: this is the first time in the history of British law that the non-therapeutic circumcision of male children has been described as a 'significant harm.' "[257]

---

256 Link to the English translation of the case: <arclaw.org/wp-content/uploads/English-Translation-of-2013-Graubunden-Swiss-Circumcision-Case.pdf>.

257 Earp BD. On the supposed distinction between culture and religion: A brief comment on Sir James Munby's decision in the matter of B and G (children). *Practical Ethics (Oxford University)*. <blog.practicalethics.ox.ac.uk/2015/02/on-the-supposed-distinction-between-

Subsequently, in April 2016, the UK's High Court of Justice (Family Division) handed down an important new decision. As in the Cologne, Germany decision, the father (a Muslim) wanted his two boys to be circumcised for religious reasons. The court refused to allow the boys to be circumcised. The court made findings that circumcision carries real risks; that nothing in Islam requires it before an age when the boys could make the decision for themselves; and that the boys, while remaining genitally intact, could fully participate in their father's Muslim community and culture and would not suffer exclusion.[258] The court held that it was in the best interests of the boys, and that it would respect their right to personal autonomy, not to allow them to be circumcised.

Courts in Europe and the UK thus appear to have reached a consensus that circumcision is harmful, and indeed that it causes significant or serious harm; that boys have the right to intact genitalia and the right to decide the fate of the foreskin for themselves; that it is in the best interests to leave their genitals alone; and that parents do not have the right to circumcise a boy, not even for religious reasons. Courts in Europe thus treat male genital cutting the same way that the U.S. Congress treated female genital cutting when it passed the anti-female genital mutilation statute.[259]

CHAPTER SUMMARY

- A German court ruled in 2012 that it is criminal assault for a physician to circumcise a boy for religious reasons, and for parents to allow it.
- Courts in Europe including the UK have made the factual findings that male genital cutting is irreversible, harmful, more harmful than some forms of female genital cutting, and that it can cause psychological harm.

culture-and-religion-a-comment-on-sir-james-munbys-decision-in-the-matter-of-b-and-g-children>.
258 Stahel P, VanderHeiden T, Kim F. Why do surgeons continue to perform unnecessary surgery? *Patient Saf Surg.* 2017;11:1. <ncbi.nlm.nih.gov/pmc/articles/PMC5234149>.
259 18 U.S.C. § 116(c) (2012). Female Genital Mutilation and Notes thereto. <law.cornell.edu/uscode/text/18/116>.

- European courts have held that boys have the right to bodily integrity and self-determination, and that the child's right to intact genitalia supersedes their parents' religious and other rights. Thus, parents do not have the right to have their son circumcised for religious or other non-medical reasons.
- These courts have also held that it is in the best interests of boys not to circumcise them.
- Courts in Europe thus treat male genital cutting the same way as the U.S. Congress treats female genital cutting in the female genital mutilation statute, as harmful and unlawful.

13 AMERICAN CASES

This chapter asks, how have courts in the United States decided circumcision cases to date?

THE STOWELL CASE

In 2000, William Stowell brought suit in federal court against the obstetrician who circumcised him as an infant and against the hospital. Stowell's mother had signed a consent form allowing the procedure, but Stowell argued that his mother's consent was legally invalid because she was heavily drugged at the time. Plaintiff's attorney David Llewellyn argued that the doctor and hospital had a fiduciary duty to ensure that the mother knew what she was signing. "And the answer is no, she did not. She does not even recall signing at all." When asked in a deposition, "And you say she wouldn't have consented or shouldn't have consented?" Stowell replied, "No, she would not have consented, nor would I have consented later on in my life." The case settled out of court.[260] Attorney Llewellyn wrote,

> William and I are very happy that we were able to resolve this case with both the hospital and the doctor. While a settlement is never an admission of liability, I believe it shows that our allegations were taken seriously. Never again can someone say that a young man who is dissatisfied with his circumcision as an infant is being frivolous when he objects to his mutilation and brings suit to obtain justice. This case should send a message to doctors that they run the risk of a lawsuit each time they circumcise an infant for non-therapeutic reasons, particularly when they rely on the hospital to obtain consent the day after birth. Social or cosmetic concerns provide no justification for harmful surgery. I would expect that this is just the first of

---

260 Transcript: <uts.edu.au/about/faculty-health/news/rise-and-fall-male-circumcision>.

many cases that will be brought by angry circumcised young men against their circumcisers.[261]

No Parental Right to Perform the Circumcision

A 2006 Washington appeals court decision, *State v. Baxter,* [262] concerned an attempt by a father – Baxter, who had no medical training – to circumcise his eight-year-old son at home with a hunting knife. The father was unable to control the boy's bleeding and called 911. The court upheld the father's conviction for criminal assault. The court reasoned that "the harm Baxter inflicted on his son triggered the State's right to impose criminal liability." The court rejected the father's defense that his god had commanded him to circumcise his son. The court acknowledged that circumcision is risky and harmful, at least when performed by a lay person without medical training. (Often physicians, nurses, and medical students are not well trained in performing circumcisions either.) It also ruled that parents without medical training do not have the right to circumcise their own son, not even for a religious reason. Importantly then, the court did not rule that parents have the unfettered religious right to circumcise their son.

No Right to Circumcise a Boy Who Objects

In *Marriage of Boldt,* [263] a long, bitter, and widely publicized 2008 Oregon Supreme Court case that primarily involved primarily custody, and secondarily circumcision and religious rights, a father who converted to Judaism wanted to have his son circumcised. The father claimed that this was required to convert him to the Jewish faith. The father argued that he had a constitutionally protected right under the freedom of religion clause

261 Doctor and Hospital Settle Circumcision Lawsuit. *Men's News Daily.* 2003-04-29. <cirp.org/news/mndnewswire04-29-03>.
262 State v. Baxter, 141 P.3d 92 (Wash. App. Div. 2006). <scholar.google.com/scholar_case?case=4914787847309781302>.
263 Marriage of Boldt, 176 P. 3d 388 (Or.; S. Ct. 2008). <scholar.google.com/scholar_case?case=15733935640861 79997>.

of the First Amendment to the U.S. Constitution to have his son circumcised.[264] Numerous powerful Jewish organizations[265] filed friends of the
court briefs supporting that claim. (Notably, as Robert Darby observed,
"At no point in their submission did they show the slightest sympathy for
the plight of the child or show any interest in his preferences in the matter."[264] In fact, even though the oral blood suction method used by some
Orthodox Jews can transmit herpes to the babies and kill them, they have
refused to abandon the practice,[266] and authorities such as the health department of the City of New York do not stop them.) The mother in turn
"testified that Misha did not want to be circumcised and was afraid to
contradict his father." Doctors Opposing Circumcision argued, correctly,
that regardless of the boy's preference, he had the right to autonomy and
to an open future bodily intact, and not to be branded as a possession of
his parents.

The U.S. physician and ethicist Douglas Diekema wrote in 2009, before the court ruled in the case, that except when medically necessary,
"circumcision should not be performed on older children and adolescents
in the face of dissent or less than enthusiastic assent." In addition, he said,
the permission of both parents should be required: boys should not be
circumcised in the face of parental disagreement.[212] Indeed, it is the rule
in Europe that both parents must consent. Dr. Diekema continued, "Whether or not she [the mother] has legal rights, I would be very reluctant to
perform an elective procedure for cultural or religious reasons without the
permission of both parents and the unambiguous assent of [the boy] himself." The court sent the case back to the trial court with instructions to
determine whether the boy wanted to be circumcised or not.

> When Misha, by now aged 14, finally got the opportunity to
> express his own opinion (at a hearing in judges' chambers in

---

264 American legal precedent confirms child's right to reject circumcision: The case of Boldt v.
   Boldt. *Circumcision Information Australia*. <circinfo.org/Boldt_case.html>.
265 American Jewish Congress; Union of Orthodox Jewish Congregations of America; American
   Jewish Committee.
266 Donaldson James S. Baby Dies of Herpes in Ritual Circumcision By Orthodox Jews. *ABC
   News*. 2012-03-09. <abcnews.go.com/Health/baby-dies-herpes-virus-ritual-circumcision-nyc-
   orthodox/story?id=15888618>.

April 2009) he made it clear that he did not wish to convert to Judaism, and *he most definitely did not want to get circumcised* or to remain with his father. Accordingly, the court issued an order that he was not to be circumcised and returned him temporarily to his father while child custody officials worked out the details of how to return him to his mother (emphasis added).[264]

The court thus implicitly rejected the argument that parents have an absolute constitutional right to have their son circumcised for religious reasons. If the father had had such an absolute right, the court could not have stopped him from exercising it. The court also implicitly recognized that it is in the best interests of boys old enough to be able to reason to let them decide the fate of their own foreskin for themselves, rather than their parents. This comports with the guideline of the American Academy of Pediatrics that children should participate in making medical decisions involving about themselves whenever possible, and with the position of the British Medical Association that boys should not be circumcised over their objection. Robert Darby wrote,

> The significance of the case is in establishing a precedent that a parent's authority to circumcise a child is not unlimited and may not even exist. Although the court took account of the boy's age (twelve), recognising that it might be difficult to get a boy of that age to lie down submissively in a doctor's surgery, it is hard to see why the principle of physical integrity would not apply to a child of any age. There [are] no obvious reasons why a child has the right to physical integrity at 12, but not at 8 years, 4 years, 6 months or 2 weeks. By the age of 12 Misha certainly knew that he wanted to keep his foreskin and was confident enough to make his views heard, and (this being the case) we may reasonably infer that if an infant or young child too young to be capable of expressing an opinion on the matter were able to do so, he would say NO, or at least ask that the operation be delayed until he was old enough to inform himself

> as to the pros, cons and harms of circumcision and make his
> own decision. ... The clear implication is that if an infant or
> child were asked if he wanted to get circumcised, and he was
> capable of giving a rational answer, the answer would be 'No
> way.' This alone is a sufficient reason why circumcision should
> not be imposed on minors.[264]

But U.S. Judges May Be Profoundly Biased in Favor of Circumcision

The *Hironimus* case, another custody dispute, went horribly wrong, and serves as a warning that any other circumcision lawsuit in the U.S. might go wrong as well. The parents entered into a separation agreement stating that the father would arrange to have the boy circumcised. The mother subsequently learned about the risks and harms of circumcision and became strenuously opposed: she wanted to protect her son from the procedure. The father then wanted to have his son circumcised all the more to spite his ex. A medical expert testified that the boy did not need to be circumcised, and that "God forbid something might go wrong," thereby informing the judge that it might. The boy said that he did not want to be circumcised. The mother spent nearly three months hiding with her then four-year-old son at a domestic violence center, and she brought suit in state court to try to stop the circumcision from taking place.

Ignoring the medical expert, the judge stated that circumcision is "very, very safe."[267] The judge was wrong: as Robert Van Howe's affidavit shows in its long list of possible complications,[268] the procedure is not safe at all, let alone very, very safe. The judge was clearly unconsciously biased in favor of circumcision. He then threw the mother in jail and ordered her to stay there until she agreed to have her son circumcised. The judge erred as the mother had the right to change her mind. After

---

267 Freeman M. Circumcision battle: Mom seeks release from jail after federal lawsuit is dismissed. *Sun Sentinel.* 2015-05-20. <sun-sentinel.com/local/palm-beach/fl-circumcision-federal-suit-dismissed-20150520-story.html>.
268 Van Howe RS. Affidavit, Appendix, Para. 13.

spending time in jail, the mother returned to court, broke down in tears, and signed the permission form.

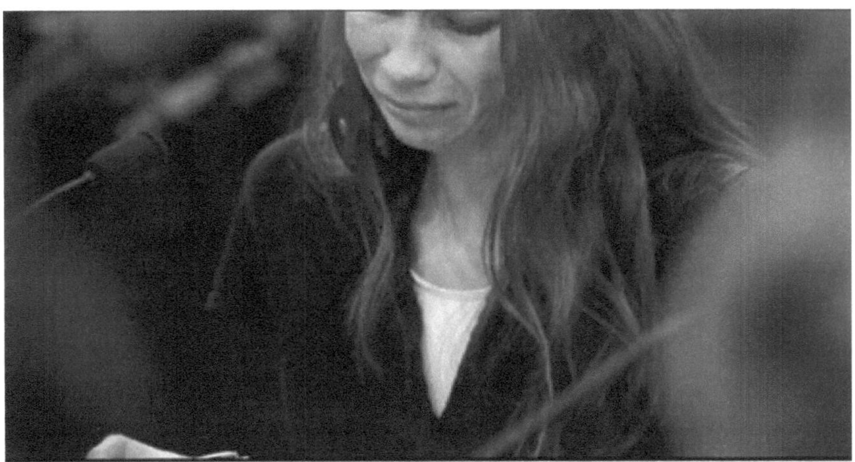

Because the mother's permission was obtained under duress ("threats, violence, constraints, or other action brought to bear on someone to do something against their will or better judgment"),[269] her permission was not legally valid. A hospital was standing by ready to circumcise the boy, even though he did not want to be circumcised and his mother did not want him to be. The father took the boy to another physician who circumcised the boy over the boy's objection, which violated his right to refuse the procedure. The physician's nurse informed me that the physician does not care whether boys (boys old enough to speak and reason) say they do not want to be circumcised or not: he circumcises them anyway. She also sent me a copy of the billing form that the physician signed. Even though a medical expert had testified that there was nothing wrong with the boy's penis, the physician falsely diagnosed the boy as suffering from "phimosis" or a tight foreskin. Otherwise, the physician would not have been paid.

The judge got this case completely wrong. He ignored the medical expert's testimony that the procedure risked complications; the mother was doing the right thing trying to protect her son from harm; the unnecessary

---

269 Definition of "duress." <google.com/search?q=duress>.

surgery violated the child's rights; and the rule is that a child's preferences must be respected.

These so-called spite circumcisions are common in custody battles. They exacerbate parental conflict, which is also harmful for the child, and they are a complete waste of judicial resources. While writing this book, other opponents of circumcision and I learned of three spite circumcisions, days before they were to take place. In one case, a friend talked the father out of it. In the second case, the mother sued, and the father decided not to litigate the matter. In the third case, the mother obtained a court order stopping the circumcision. Astonishingly, the hospital planned to go ahead with it anyway. The mother went to the hospital and gave them a copy of the court order, but the hospital refused to talk to her. I called the hospital's risk management department and reached the right person, who refused to talk to me and hung up on me. When I asked the mother whether she was able to save her son, she wrote, "Unfortunately not. I cried for literally 8 hours when I found out." Although the hospital mentioned above ultimately backed down in the face of the threat of a lawsuit for violating a court order, the father found another physician to circumcise the boy, as had happened in the *Hironimus* case. Given that the hospital was planning to circumcise the boy despite a court order forbidding it, and that it only relented at the last minute after being threatened with a lawsuit, the conclusion seems inescapable that some hospitals are hell bent on circumcising every boy they can. Of course, there is an endless supply of newborn boys for them to circumcise.

A Pending Lawsuit Accuses the AAP of Fraud in 1989

A lawsuit is pending in federal court in New Jersey, brought by a man injured by circumcision and his parents, accusinging the American Academy of Pediatrics of having issued fraudulent circumcision guidelines in 1989. The AAP has moved to dismiss the case, the plaintiffs have opposed the motion to dismiss, and a ruling on the motion is pending. If the plaintiffs prevail, it will be a huge though interim victory in circumcision litigation; and if they lose, they are likely to appeal the decision.

- Courts in the U.S. have erred in not ruling yet that male genital cutting is harmful and unlawful.
- U.S. courts are moving in the right direction, however, in ruling that parents do not have the unfettered right to elect to have their son circumcised for religious reasons, and in deciding implicitly that boys old enough to reason should be able to decide the fate of the foreskin for themselves.
- A pending suit accusing the AAP of having issued fraudulent circumcision guidelines in 1989 might shake up the industry if it succeeds.
- More lawsuits arising from the practice are coming to the USA.

This Part, the heart of the book, shows how circumcision is a complex 150 year old multibillion dollar per year fraud. Chapter 14 shows that the past is prelude to the present. Chapter 15 shows that physicians and hospitals have several undisclosed conflicts of interest and motives to commit fraud. Chapter 16 discusses the elements of fraud. Chapter 17 shows how hospitals and medical groups use fraudulent advertising and marketing to promote circumcision. Chapter 18 shows how physicians and nurses engage in fraudulent conduct in hospitals. Chapter 19 shows how physicians and nurses make frivolous and hence fraudulent claims. Chapter 20 shows how physicians and their trade associations defraud boys, men, and their parents by making the false medical claim that genital cutting is not bad for health. Chapter 21 shows how physicians and their trade associations defraud boys, men, and their parents by making the false medical claim that genital cutting is good for health. Chapter 22 shows how physicians and their trade associations make the false and fraudulent legal claim that physicians are allowed to operate on a healthy child, and to take orders from parents to do so. Chapter 23 shows how physicians and hospitals use fraudulent consent forms. Chapter 24 shows how they use fraudulent diagnoses and how physicians and their trade associations defraud the federal and state Medicaid program. Chapter 25 shows how circumcision also constitutes so-called constructive or equitable fraud. Chapter 26 shows how physicians and the American Academy of Pediatrics advance frivolous and hence fraudulent defenses in lawsuit and sometimes retaliate against the plaintiff.

14   THE PAST AS PRELUDE TO THE PRESENT

Given the brutal history of genital cutting or mutilation, and the immense suffering that it has caused worldwide for thousands of years, one would have expected that physicians worldwide would refuse to perform the operation and would warn against it. Physicians in most developed countries do not circumcise healthy boys, and initially physicians in the United Kingdom and the United States did not either. As Laura Carpenter observed, "[f]or centuries, Britons and their North American cousins viewed male circumcision as a Jewish or Muslim religious ritual at best and a disfiguring, heathen practice at worst."[76] Several national and international medical organizations recommend against it. For example, in 1999 the Australasian Association of Paediatric Surgeons called it unnecessary and inappropriate to remove the prepuce.[270] And in 2010, The Royal Dutch Medical Association condemned the practice and advised its member physicians, who for the most part refuse to perform the operation, to use their best efforts to deter parents from electing to have their son circumcised.

The question thus arises, how did physicians in the United States become outliers in circumcising healthy boys? How were they able to turn violence into a profitable industry? The short answer is, by aggressively promoting it while not telling Americans the truth about it. As will be seen, they use the same unfair and deceptive practices as in the past to this day, and when those fail, they invent new ones.

MASTURBATION HYSTERIA

Just as boys' and girls' genitals were cut in ancient times to control their sexuality, Gollaher recounts how during the mid-19th to early 20th centuries, the Victorian era, boys were circumcised to correct a diverse range of perceived sexual problems, including "sexual unrest," impotence, homosexuality, and especially the "vile habit of masturbation."[46] In 1758, Samuel Auguste Tissot wrote a treatise on Onanism, the disorders produced by masturbation, which led to the nineteenth century's invective

---

270 AAPS: Guidelines for Circumcision. <cirp.org/library/statements/aaps>.

against that perceived vice. Darby recounts, "it has been widely accepted by medical historians since the 1950s that discouraging masturbation was a major reason why doctors, educationists and childcare experts sought to introduce widespread circumcision of both boys and girls in the nineteenth century, a campaign which was successful in the former case, unsuccessful in the latter."[32] Thus, physicians in English speaking countries including the United States circumcised both boys and girls in an effort to suppress their sexuality.[32] Dr. John Harvey Kellogg, the inventor of Kellogg's corn flakes, promoted circumcision as a cure for masturbation. "A remedy which is almost always successful in small boys is circumcision. The operation should be performed by a surgeon without administering an anesthetic, as the brief pain attending the operation will have a salutary effect upon the mind." Thus, physicians during the Victorian era intentionally caused pain to perfectly healthy boys, and girls.

Darby states that "surgical and pharmacological methods of preventing masturbation were certainly widespread." Brutal and punitive treatments, "introduced in the second half of the nineteenth century included chastity belts and genital infibulation for both sexes, and spiked collars to wrap around the penis of boys afflicted by nocturnal emissions." (Female infibulation is the practice of excising the clitoris and labia of a girl or woman and stitching together the edges of the vulva to prevent sexual intercourse.)[271] Other methods included "castration and severing the dorsal nerve of the penis in males; and clitoridectomy and ovariotomy in females." These methods, performed without anesthetic, were unspeakably cruel, and not surprisingly they harmed the boys and girls psychologically. A 1930 study of children with psychological and behavioural problems reported that "a high proportion of the boys had been threatened with mutilating operations on their penis if they masturbated."

Ironically, circumcised men masturbate more frequently than men with a foreskin,[272] another example of the ways that circumcision can change a male's sex life. Of course, nocturnal emissions and masturbation are normal, and masturbation proved to be popular. In the modern era, in

271 Definition of "infibulation." <google.com/search?q=infibulation>.
272 Laumann, EO, Masi CM, Zuckerman EW. Circumcision in the United States: Prevalence, Prophylactic Effects, and Sexual Practice. *JAMA*. 1997;277(13):1052-7. <cirp.org/library/general/laumann>.

1999, the United Kingdom encouraged it.[273] The claim that circumcision prevented it appealed to parents during the Victorian era in Great Britain, however, and gave a jump start to the practice in the puritanical United States. It was unacceptable that American physicians punished boys, sometimes severely, for masturbating.

EARLY FALSE MEDICAL CLAIMS: A CURE IN SEARCH FOR A DISEASE

Robert Darby states that the "concept of circumcision as a preventive, and then routine, procedure emerged in the mid-nineteenth century."[32] Physicians circumcised boys only in Great Britain – where it lasted from the 1870s to the late 1940s – and in the other English-speaking countries: Canada, Australia, New Zealand, and the United States.

According to David Gollaher,[32] physicians claimed that the foreskin is not merely dirty but vulgar and the cause of a variety of diseases. Sarah Waldeck writes, "The penis was seen as an especially virulent source of contamination."[50] As one example of this demonization of the foreskin, the American medical scholar G. N. Weiss stated that "over the millennia the male's preputial cavity has acted as a cesspool for infectious agents transmitting disease."[274]

Lewis Sayre, a highly respected English physician, hypothesized in 1870 that the prepuce caused irritability in children, restless sleep, bad digestion, and hip problems. He circumcised boys in an insane asylum seeking a cure for lunacy. He also claimed that the operation helped cure epilepsy, hernia, and insanity of the muscles.[46] In addition, Sayre "revived the mutilating procedure of clitoridectomy, with the clitoris subjected to a variety of surgeries, manipulations, and chemical preparations."[46]

David Gollaher notes that female genital surgeries, like male genital surgeries, continued in the United States long after they had fallen out of favor in Europe. Thus, the U.S. was slow and an outlier in abandoning female genital cutting, just as it is slow and an outlier today in refusing to abandon male genital cutting today. Physicians also circumcised boys in

---

273 Treptow C. U.K. Government Encourages Teen Masturbation? *ABC News.* 2009-07-13. <abcnews.go.com/Health/MindMoodNews/story?id=8072314&page=1>.

274 International Coalition for Genital Integrity circumcision timeline here with citations to scientific articles. <icgi.org/medicalization>.

an unsuccessful effort to cure syphilis,[46] the frightening sexually transmitted disease of the day. This presages the false claim by the American Academy of Pediatrics in 2012 that it prevents the spread of our most current alarming sexually transmitted disease: HIV.

Edward Wallerstein called Dr. P. C. Remondino the most prolific enumerator of health benefits. In 1891 this physician claimed that the surgery prevented or cured about one hundred ailments, including alcoholism, epilepsy, asthma, enuresis, hernia, gout, rectal prolapse, rheumatism, and kidney disease, among many others. The book was reprinted in 1974 without change.[89] Doctor Remondino also argued that the invention of clothes, which protect the glans in its thorny passage through life, made the foreskin superfluous.[275] In David Gollaher's opinion, "Remondino's 'facts' appear to be a rambling, slapdash collection of folklore, conjecture, opinion, and pseudoscience."

Although Remondino was especially prolific in advancing different rationales for circumcision, he was by no means alone in doing so. Physicians erroneously claimed under medical theories circulating at the time that removing the foreskin cured or prevented more than 100 diseases.[275] These included epilepsy,[276] eye problems,[277] paralysis,[278] and tuberculosis.[279] One physician went so far as to claim that it prevented, "nearly all physical and mental illness[es]."[280] A timeline shows that as a result of these claims, the circumcision rate in the United States rose from essentially zero in the mid to late 1800s to the high 80% range by the mid-1900s.

Granted, these were the early pre-scientific days of medicine, and likely some physicians such as Sayre believed their false medical claims to be true. On the other hand, in the early days of medicine, before physi-

---

275 International Coalition for Genital Integrity circumcision timeline here with citations to scientific articles. <icgi.org/medicalization>.

276 Sayre LA, Detmold JC, Hutchinson R. Circumcision versus epilepsy, etc., Transcription of the New York Pathological Society meeting of June 8, 1870. *Med Record.* 1870-07-15;5(10):231-4.

277 Landesberg M. On affections of the eye caused by masturbation. *Med Bull.* 1881-04;3(4):79-81.

278 Sayre LA. Partial paralysis from reflex irritation, caused by congenital phimosis and adherent prepuce. *Transactions of the AMA.* 1870;21:205-11.

279 Wolbarst AL. Universal circumcision as a sanitary measure. *JAMA.* 1914-01-10;62(2):92-7.

280 Miller RL, Snyder DC. Immediate circumcision of the newborn male. *Am J Obstet Gynecol.* 1953-01;6(1):1-11.

cians were licensed and became subject to the rules of medical ethics, some physicians were quacks peddling cures they knew to be fake (just as some lawyers were shysters). The fact that physicians advanced new reasons for the practice whenever the last reason was proven false, however, more than one hundred times, strongly suggests that many of the physicians advanced their reasons in bad faith and with intent to deceive parents or the public about the practice. Furthermore, "When you look through history, you see that whatever the scary disease of the generation was, that was the one that circumcision would help prevent. During the 20th century, syphilis was the scary disease; later it was cancer; and today it is HIV."[281]

Moreover, it is the classic and ridiculous claim of quacks selling useless tonics or "snake oil" to assert that a potion or procedure prevents most or all diseases. Since the late 1800s, physicians and American medical associations have claimed that circumcision prevents, cures, or reduces the risk of so many diseases that it might be impossible for anyone to find them all. Thus, circumcision in the "old days" was quack medicine, supported by junk science, and sometimes if not often a fraud.

David Gollaher also recounts how physicians suggested circumcision to parents immediately after the birth of a son, claiming that the operation was simple, safe, and reduced the infant's chances of becoming infected with the deadly and fearsome diseases of childhood. As discussed below, physicians in the U.S. have used the same and other false medical claims and scare tactics to promote the practice to this day. A 1912 treatise claimed that "Parents who do not have an early circumcision performed on their boys are almost criminally negligent."[282] Ironically, as discussed in Chapter 10 (The Perfect Crime), it is the physicians who are committing the crime.

By demonizing the prepuce, by making false claims about the medical benefits of male genital cutting, by arguing that the foreskin was a "constricting, unnatural band," by falsely claiming that male genital cutting is painless, and by not evaluating its risks,[46] physicians in the U.S. succeed-

281 Eli Ungar-Sargon, who made a film, "Cut," that questions circumcision, quoted in: Rabin RC. The Latest Fight Over the Foreskin. *NY Times.* 2009-07-29.

282 Lydston GF. Impotence and sterility. Riverton Press. 1917; p. 89. <books.google.de/books? id=_3y7BeWWxQgC>.

ed in turning a painful religious rite and cultural practice into a routine procedure perceived to be medicine, when it is still violence masquerading as medicine.

Darby insightfully describes the procedure as a "surgical temptation,"[283] one which physicians have manifestly been unable to resist for the past one hundred and fifty years. It is good for profits; parents know little or nothing about it and physicians do not enlighten them; and the babies and older boys are powerless to prevent it. As a result, circumcision "became ingrained in the collective medical consciousness, appearing too obviously salubrious to warrant formal analysis of benefits, harms, costs, and outcomes."[46] David Gollaher observed frighteningly that, "By all indications, the procedure was done with little thought."[46]

EARLY FALSE DIAGNOSES

Physicians also falsely diagnosed "redundant foreskin," meaning a long foreskin, as being a medical condition requiring removal. Of course, just as the length of all parts of different people's bodies vary in length, so does the length of the foreskin of boys' penises. One that overlaps the glans penis is perfectly normal. Rather than being a bad thing, as these physicians claimed, having more foreskin is a good thing as it is replete with nerves and highly erogenous.

In addition, physicians have for many years diagnosed "phimosis" or a tight foreskin as a reason to circumcise. The physician Lewis Sayre claimed that a tight foreskin, as well as a long foreskin, can cause complications and therefore, "it is always good surgery to correct this deformity... as a precautionary measure, even though no symptoms have as yet presented themselves."[46] Physicians thus portrayed a normal, tight foreskin as a pathological condition needing treatment. At birth, however, the foreskin firmly adheres to the glans penis, like nails to a nail bed. The two naturally separate but sometimes not until puberty.[284] I was shocked to learn that as a result, physicians must use a blunt instrument to force

283 Darby RJL. *A Surgical Temptation: the Demonization of the Foreskin and the Rise of Circumcision in Britain.* <amazon.com/dp/0226136450>.
284 Circumcision Information Resource Center. Normal Development of the Prepuce: Birth Through Age 18. With citations to scientific authorities. <cirp.org/library/normal>.

the foreskin apart from the glans. Being circumcised is therefore analogous to having one's nails pulled out, which is widely viewed as a form of torture, except that nails grow back whereas the foreskin does not. Like a long foreskin, then, a tight foreskin is normal and not a birth defect. Moreover, even a pathologically tight foreskin can be treated with stretching and steroids. The diagnosis of phimosis was a scam. As discussed in Chapter 24 (Fraudulent Diagnoses and Medicaid Fraud), lacking a valid diagnosis to operate on healthy older boys, physicians often use the false diagnosis of phimosis to this day.

EARLY FRIVOLOUS CLAIMS

By the mid-1900s, physicians were also giving parents a wide variety of plainly frivolous reasons to elect circumcision, which they would not have done had they been able to justify it on medical grounds. By contrast, physicians do not give adults frivolous reasons for hip surgery; and if they did, the reasons would be rejected outright as absurd.

For example, physicians have claimed that the circumcised penis is aesthetically superior;[83] that being circumcised saves boy from being embarrassed in the locker room;[285] that it is difficult to clean the foreskin[286] (even though soap has been invented); or simply that it is "better" for boys to be circumcised, without saying why. As mentioned, physicians also claimed that the foreskin is no longer needed now that we have clothes.

One mother told me that an obstetrician came to circumcise her newborn son, told her and her husband nothing about circumcision, and seemed irate that they had not signed the circumcision consent form. The father told the OB, "The AAP [American Academy of Pediatrics] said it is not medically necessary," which the OB should have been telling the father. "The only thing the OB could say was 'Well, everybody wants one.' "[287] This is another false and frivolous claim. Not all parents want

285 Preston EN. Whither the Foreskin? A Consideration of Routine Neonatal Circumcision. *JAMA.* 1970;213:1853-54.
286 1975 AAP Statement. "Circumcision ... eliminates much of the need for careful penile hygiene." <cirp.org/library/statements/aap/#a1975>.
287 Email communication. 2021-08-17.

one, and more importantly, boys and men do not want one. Doctors and hospitals want them.

The American Academy of Pediatrics even made the ridiculous claims in 1975 that "[f]actors such as climate, the social and emotional reaction of prospective parents to penile cleansing, and the ability to understand and facilitate good hygiene, etc. should be taken into account when recommending whether circumcision should be performed."[286] According to the AAP, then, when deciding whether to circumcise a boy, the physician should consider the weather where one lives, the parents' intelligence, and their feelings about cleaning the foreskin. Lay people trust physicians so much that they believe even ludicrous claims like these.

Acknowledged that Not Medically Justified

Largely Abandoned By Other English-Speaking Countries

In a landmark paper in 1949,[83] the British physician Douglas Gairdner issued a strong warning against removing the foreskin. Gairdner wrote that in ancient times, male circumcision was often associated with analogous sexual mutilations of the female. Although circumcision was one of the most common operations in Great Britain, it had been accorded the least critical consideration, and little was known about the anatomy or function of the foreskin or the hazards of the operation; a frightening thought for the boys being subjected to it. He set out to remedy the situation through scientific analysis.

Gairdner reported that the few genitally intact men he had spoken with were emphatic that they considered it to be to their advantage to have a foreskin. That led him to conclude that "few uncircumcised men have cause to regret their state." As stated above, even though about 85% of males in the U.S. were circumcised in 1965,[272] genitally intact men rarely volunteered to be circumcised then, nor do they now. In short, Gairdner concluded that males who have a foreskin value it and do not want to part with it.

Gairdner observed that in early childhood, the foreskin adheres to the glans penis, and it separates over time. Thus, he showed that phimosis or a tight foreskin is usually normal and not a valid reason to circumcise a boy, even though it is often the diagnosis that physicians use. He then noted that like any other operation, circumcision risks complications, including meatal ulceration, sometimes requiring additional hospitalization and treatment. Gairdner further discovered that circumcision is sometimes fatal, even when performed in hospitals, due to infection, hemorrhage, and anemia, to which young children are particularly susceptible, and anesthetic deaths.

He stated that the evidence does not warrant universal circumcision as a prophylactic (a preventative measure) against venereal infection, and that good hygiene would confer the same immunity as being circumcised from penile cancer (the disease du jour). So long as the prepuce is kept clean, most of the tens of thousands of circumcisions performed annually in Great Britain each year could be avoided, along with meatal ulceration, unnecessary deaths, much parental anxiety, and an appreciable amount of the time of doctors and nurses.

Gairdner also dismissed some of the reasons advanced for circumcision as trivial, such as "difficulties in keeping the uncircumcised parts clean, or the supposed aesthetic or erotic superiority of the shorn member." After critically examining, "[t]he many and varied reasons commonly advanced for circumcising infants," Gairdner concluded that none were convincing, and that "the prepuce of the young infant should therefore be left in its natural state."[83]

The following year, in 1950, the British National Health Service dropped circumcision from its list of covered services. Parents who wanted their sons circumcised were required to pay a surgical fee for it, and most parents were unwilling to do so. As a result, as David Gollaher reports, the circumcision rate plummeted from 50% of working-class and 85% of upper-class Englishmen before World War II, to less than one half of 1% in the 1960s.[46] Thereafter, British Commonwealth countries also stopped paying for it, and circumcision rates in those countries dramatically declined, as they had in Great Britain.[288] This did not result in an outbreak of the diseases that physicians had introduced circumcision to prevent.

---

288 Wallerstein E. Circumcision: the uniquely American medical enigma. See note #89: "the practice has virtually been abandoned."

New Zealand largely gave up the practice in the 1960s, while circumcision rates fell in Australia and Canada beginning in the 1970s.[32] In the 1950s, the circumcision rate in Australia was approximately 80%, whereas today it is about 20%.[289]

Not Medically Justified

As discussed, it is rare for physicians to circumcise boys in the developed world outside of the United States, South Korea (which the U.S. occupied), and Israel, where boys are circumcised for religious reasons. Physicians in other parts of the English-speaking world have largely abandoned the practice. In stark contrast, in the United States by 1980, the circumcision rate was 88%.[89] As Wallerstein observed, "The United States stands alone as the only country in the world in which the majority of newborn males are circumcised [by physicians], purportedly for health reasons."[89]

A 1969 article in *The New England Journal of Medicine* concluded, however, that "[T]here was insufficient evidence to justify any surgery as a preventive measure," and that "cutting in the absence of disease violated the most cherished tenet of medical ethics, *primum non nocere* ("First, Do No Harm")."[46] In 1971, another pediatrician concluded after reviewing the medical literature that "none of the substantial medical benefits associated with it – primarily prevention of sexually transmitted diseases and cancers of the penis and prostate – could withstand scrutiny."[46] The highly respected *New England Journal* concluded that "circumcision is a beautification comparable to rhinoplasty [a nose job]": i.e., it is *cosmetic surgery,* albeit without the consent of the person whose body is being modified.

A 1978 article in the *American Journal of Obstetrics and Gynecology* stated that circumcision enthusiasts used illogical bases for patient selection, lack of informed consent, disregard for pain, unskilled surgeons, and unclear clinical objectives. The article concluded that "Clinicians ought to use techniques only when certain that they do good … In clinical practice physicians should not have to prove that techniques are not danger-

289 abc.net.au/science/articles/2012/08/27/3576889.htm

ous."[290,46] The best-selling medical author Benjamin Spock, who had originally endorsed circumcision, also concluded that the operation seemed "unnecessary and at least mildly dangerous"[46] (actually it is very dangerous, whereas leaving the foreskin alone involves no risk).

Importantly, as mentioned above, the American Academy of Pediatrics has never recommended circumcision either. In 1971, it issued its first circumcision policy guideline stating simply, "There are no valid medical indications for circumcision in the neonatal period."[285] In medicine, an indication is a valid medical reason to use a certain procedure or surgery to treat a medical condition. Thus, the AAP acknowledged in 1971, as remains true today, that there is no valid medical reason to circumcise any newborn boy, as physicians in the U.S. have done more than one hundred million times since the late 1800s. In 1977, the AAP stated that circumcision is not an essential component of health care,[291] acknowledging that it is not medically necessary. In 1989 and 1999, although the Academy claimed that newborn male circumcision has potential health benefits and advantages, it acknowledged that it also has disadvantages and risks, and it did not assert that the potential health benefits outweigh the disadvantages and risks. To justify an operation, a physician needs to show – at a minimum – not only that the patient needs the operation, but also that the operation is likely to do more good than harm. The AAP also stated in 1999 that "behavioral factors appear to be far more important than circumcision status" in causing sexually transmitted diseases including HIV.

In 1999, the American Medical Association concluded that circumcision is *not medically justified,*[292] which is what the Harvard physician told me in 1987. Specifically, the AMA cited a model of decision making concluding that "the incidence of UTI would have to be substantially higher in circumcised males to justify circumcision as a preventive measure against this condition." Because penile cancer "is rare and occurs

290 Grimes A. Routine Circumcision of the Newborn Infant: A Reappraisal. *Am J Obstetrics & Gynecology.* 1978-01-15;130(2):125-9. <cirp.org/library/general/grimes>.

291 Oh W, Merenstein G. 1997 AAP Statement. Fourth Edition of the Guidelines for Perinatal Care: Summary of Changes. *Pediatrics.* 1997;100:1021. <cirp.org/library/statements/aap/#a1977>.

292 1999 AMA Statement. "existing scientific evidence demonstrates potential medical benefits of newborn male circumcision; however, these data are not sufficient to recommend routine neonatal circumcision" <cirp.org/library/statements/ama2000>.

later in life, the use of circumcision as a preventive practice is not justi-fied." The AMA also stated, as did the AAP the same year, that because "behavioral factors are far more important risk factors for acquisition of HIV and other sexually transmitted diseases than circumcision status, *circumcision cannot responsibly be viewed as protecting against such diseases* (emphasis added)."[292] Thus, American medical associations knew by 1999 at the latest that circumcision is not medically justified. It had a duty at that time to advise its member physicians to abandon the practice.

Accusation of Negligence and Possible Fraud by the AAP in 1989 and 1999

In 1989 and 1999, the American Academy of Pediatrics revised its cir-cumcision guidelines. In 1999, the legal scholar Matthew Giannetti ana-lyzed them and found that they were biased in favor of circumcision and deeply flawed. He asserted that they exposed the AAP to trade association liability for scientific misconduct for negligence and possibly also for intentional fraud.

Continuing the longstanding practice of claiming that circumcision prevents a new disease whenever the last claim had been disproved, in 1989 the AAP advanced another new justification, namely that new evi-dence showed that the procedure had the potential medical benefit of lower rates of urinary tract infections (UTIs) among circumcised infants. The studies were biased and flawed, however; and regardless, the appro-priate treatment for UTIs is antibiotics, which are readily available in developed countries, inexpensive, and highly effective. The 1989 report understated pain, calling it, "transient and disappear[ing] within 24 hours after surgery," when pain continues thereafter, and usually it is not treat-ed. The AAP also ignored the warnings about the unknown long-term effects of pain around the newborn period. Giannetti found it shocking that the AAP ignored research showing that circumcision causes long-term behavioral changes.

Giannetti discussed how in 1984 the AAP had issued a brochure, *Care of the Uncircumcised Penis,* describing the protective function of the foreskin in shielding the head of the penis from irritation and infection, and the adverse consequences of its loss after circumcision, namely the risk of infection and narrowing of the urethral opening, sometimes requiring additional surgery or surgeries. The psychologist Dr. Ronald Goldman asked the AAP in writing eight times why it had removed this useful information from the pamphlet, and he suggested that the information be included in the brochure again. The AAP never gave him a satisfactory explanation why it had removed the information or why it had not put the information back in again.[293] Giannetti charitably concluded that the AAP had, "displayed a bias in favor of circumcision by altering its brochure for parents." The incident shows that the AAP knew about this risk, disclosed it at one time, and then stopped disclosing it. It can be inferred that the AAP decided that it no longer wanted parents to know that the foreskin protects the glans for life, or that circumcision can cause infection and narrowing of the urethral opening, because if parents knew that information, they might say "no" to circumcision. In fact, as recounted in the Prologue, when my son was born, and the physician did disclose that information to me, I considered that to be a a reason to decline the offered procedure.) Giannetti also wrote, "The AAP also displayed bias in omitting the higher prevalence of meatitis and non-specific urethritis in circumcised men." The only reason why the AAP would not mention those risks is that it did not want parents and the public to know about them either.

In 1949, Douglas Gairdner wrote that little was known about the hazards of the operation. Astonishingly, in 1989, forty years later, the AAP, "still could not authoritatively cite a complication rate for circumcision." The 1989 AAP report stated that circumcision has disadvantages and potential medical benefits, but it did not weigh the two, or claim that the benefits outweigh the disadvantages, as physicians are required to determine before performing a procedure. The AAP concluded that "these data are not sufficient to recommend routine neonatal circumcision." This violates the rule that physicians must recommend the optimal treatment for each patient. Giannetti observed that the AAP had failed in its duty to

---

293 Goldman R. AAP Pamphlet "Care of the Uncircumcised Penis" Included Foreskin Functions. 1996-10-01. <circumcision.org/aap-pamphlet-care-of-the-uncircumcised-penis-included-foreskin-functions>.

justify circumcision as a preventive medical procedure. Instead, the AAP had "left the decision to the 'cultural' desires of parents."

Matthew Giannetti cited a ground-breaking 1996 New Jersey Supreme Court decision, *Snyder v. American Association of Blood Banks,* [294] in arguing that the AAP faced legal claims as a trade association. In *Snyder*, the plaintiff contracted AIDS from a transfusion with contaminated blood. The court stated that "[b]y words and conduct, the AABB [American Association of Blood Banks] invited blood banks, hospitals, and patients to rely on the AABB's recommended procedures." The guidelines did not adopt a better testing procedure that likely would have detected HIV and have prevented the plaintiff from contracting it. Giannetti argued that, like the blood banks, the AAP could be held liable as a trade association for having issued negligent and possibly fraudulent circumcision guidelines in 1989 and 1999.

> The paramount responsibility of the AAP is promoting the health of children. As the AAP's own mission explains the organization's purpose, it is 'to obtain optimal physical, mental, and social health and wellbeing for all infants, children, adolescents and young adults.' The AAP's mission is not to satisfy the extraneous concerns of parental or physician choices in 'esthetics, religion, cultural attitudes, social pressures, and tradition.' The AAP should inform the public of its failure to find clear medical benefits from this surgery, while fully disclosing the risk of adverse outcomes known to occur. *In sum it should discontinue the classification of this surgery as acceptable medical care for infant boys* (emphasis added).[295]

That is to say, the AAP has a duty to stop claiming that circumcision is medicine or an acceptable medical practice. One would have expected the AAP to have defended itself against Giannetti's claim that its guidelines

---

294 Snyder v. American Ass'n of Blood Banks, 676 A. 2d 1036 (NJ: S. Ct. 1996).
<scholar.google.com/scholar_case?case=7059830066439806422>.
295 Giannetti MR. Circumcision and the American Academy of Pediatrics: Should Scientific Misconduct Result in Trade Association Liability? *Iowa Law Review.* 2000-05;85(4);1507-68.
<cirp.org/library/legal/giannetti/04.html>

were negligent and possibly fraudulent, but it did not. It can be inferred that the AAP did not want the American public to know about these accusations, and that it did not have a convincing defense. Some of Giannetti's criticisms of the AAP's 1989 and 1999 guidelines also apply to AAP's most recent 2012 guidelines. For example, the AAP still does not know the extent of the risk of complications decades later.

Deeply Embedded and Self-Perpetuating Cultural Norm

In 2003, Sarah Waldeck wrote an insightful article[44] about how social or cultural norms regulate social behavior, establish what constitutes appropriate conduct, color every aspect of how people make decisions and behave, and importantly, thereby cause us to "persist in our beliefs in ways that are normatively indefensible." Waldeck considered male circumcision to be the quintessential example of such a norm. At one end of the spectrum, some tribes practice skin stripping – the harshest form of male genital cutting – near puberty, and to members of those tribes, that is the cultural norm and tradition. In Islamic culture, it is the norm to circumcise boys as a rite of passage around age ten or puberty, while "uncircumcised people are 'abnormal' and seen as lacking something."[47] (Of course, the foreskin is normal and what is abnormal from the evolutionary, historic, and global perspective is for a male not to have one.) South Korean boys in turn are circumcised during late elementary school. Waldeck states that the thought of having a boy circumcised at ten years old or puberty might make an American wince, but South Koreans have the same response to the practice in the U.S. of circumcising boys shortly after they are born. At the other end of the spectrum, in Sweden, "routine circumcision is non-existent and widely perceived as an assault on the child."

Waldeck discusses how "history matters" in understanding the upward trajectory of neonatal circumcision in the United States in the late 1800s to the early to mid-1900s. The practice of physicians associating the foreskin with many diseases and promoting it as preventative medicine, in the absence of a disorder, coincided with an increase in the number of hospitals and the number of boys born in hospitals rather than at home. This made circumcision more convenient and safer, though as will be seen, still not safe. "Over time, the medical profession came to understand that circumcision neither prevented masturbation nor provided the panoply of benefits that Sayre and others had presumed it would." Nonetheless, doctors in the U.S. continued to promote the practice opportunistically and to make unsustainable arguments in favor of it.

As a result, the practice became ubiquitous and routine in the U.S. and ingrained in the collective consciousness as medicine, "appearing too obviously salubrious to warrant formal analysis of benefits, harms, costs, and outcomes."[38] It also became a "deeply internalized norm of good parenting," even though "usual conceptions of acting in a child's best interest do not include having him undergo [an unnecessary] surgery that has associated risks and is not medically warranted." Moreover, once most fathers were circumcised, physicians asked the parents whether they want their son's penis to "look like" the father's penis. This question results in many parents electing to have their son circumcised. Thus, the practice became self-perpetuating, and it remains so in the U.S. to this day. In fact, even though the 2012 American Academy of Pediatrics circumcision guidelines automatically expired in 2017, the AAP does not need to continue to issue any more guidelines for Americans to believe that circumcision is medicine. On the other hand, the circumcision rate in the U.S. is about 55% today. If it declines to below 50%, one generation later, more parents will want their son's penis to be genitally intact than circumcised.

CHAPTER SUMMARY

- Physicians introduced circumcision to the U.S. by falsely claiming that it prevented masturbation, which appealed to parents during the puritanical era. They demonized the foreskin as dirty and as the cause of infections. They also falsely claimed that the procedure prevented or cured more than one hundred diseases and even all diseases, the classic claims of medical quacks selling "snake oil."
- They falsely portrayed circumcision as the simple, painless, harmless snip of a useless piece of skin.

- They used false diagnoses such as "long foreskin" and "tight foreskin," both of which are normal.
- They made specious or frivolous claims in favor of the practice, such as that it is difficult to clean the foreskin or that boys would be embarrassed in the locker room if their penis looks different.
- They also took unfair advantage of parents in the hospital, such as by unlawfully circumcising boys without the parents' permission, which was an unlawful battery.
- American medical associations acknowledged in 1971 that there is no medical indication or need to circumcise newborn boys, and the AMA stated in 1999 that the practice is not medically justified.
- In 1999, a legal scholar accused the AAP of having issued possibly fraudulent guidelines in 1989 and 1999 to maintain physicians' profits, and the AAP did not respond to or refute the accusations.
- As a result of these various unfair and deceptive practices, the American medical profession caused circumcision to become a deeply embedded and self-perpetuating cultural norm in the United States.

15   Undisclosed Conflicts of Interest and Motives to Defraud

As shown in Chapter 7 (Physicians' Duties), physicians who circumcise and the American Academy of Pediatrics representing them have a legal and ethical duty to be completely loyal, honest, and fair to patients and their legal representatives. This requires that they disclose any conflict of interest. Conflicts can be pernicious[296] as they can cause the physician to act in his or her own best interests rather than in the best interests of the physician's patient. The AAP recognizes the importance of disclosing conflicts of interest because when it solicited public comments on its 2012 circumcision guidelines, it required those who made comments to disclose their conflicts of interest, if any. Physicians who circumcise and the AAP have serious and substantial conflicts of interest in favor of the practice, or motives to defraud, that they do not disclose to parents or the American public.

Financial

Since physicians are not allowed to perform unnecessary surgery without consent, they are not allowed to charge a fee for performing it. Billing for unnecessary surgery other than cosmetic surgery places the physician's own financial interests above the welfare of his or her patient.[196] (Notably, healthy boys do not even meet the definition of a "patient," namely "a person receiving medical treatment." Nor does circumcision meet the definition of "surgery," namely using manual and instrumental techniques on a person to treat pathological condition such as a disease or injury.)

Three surgeons admit that surgeons often perform unnecessary surgery for *personal financial gain.*[258] A June 22, 1987, article in the *Boston Globe* quoted Thomas Wiswell, M.D. as having said, "I have some good friends who are obstetricians outside the military, and they look at a foreskin and almost see a $125 price tag on it. Each one is that much money. Heck, if you do 10 a week, that's over $1,000 a week, and they don't take

---

296 Volkov M.The Pernicious Effect of Conflicts of Interest. *JD Supra.* 2018-06-20. <jdsupra.com/legalnews/the-pernicious-effect-of-conflicts-of-80647>.

that much time."[297] (Adjusted for inflation, $1,000 per week or $52,000 per year in 1987 is worth $127,230 in 2021.) The income can help a physician pay for college or put a fancier car in the driveway. What a great business model! There is an endless supply of newborn boys unable to refuse the operation; physicians do not need to bother making a diagnosis; it is easy to persuade parents to say "yes" (for example just say "it's better"), and if the parents say "no," just badger them until they say "yes". Only physicians can perform operations in hospitals, so there is no competition; the work is quick and easy; do not bother following up after the operation to see what harm you have caused; and the pay is good.

How large, then, is the incentive for physicians and hospitals to keep circumcising healthy boys? According to the AAP in a confidential memorandum to its member pediatricians in 2012, the average cost of one is "upwards of $1,750" when hospital fees, supplies, and anesthesia [when used] are considered.[298] Assuming that physicians in the U.S. currently circumcise 1.5 million healthy boys per year, as Intact America estimates, that adds up to a continuing income stream of up to $2.6 billion per year, according to the AAP's own numbers.

In addition, undisclosed to parents, pediatric urologists are kept busy trying to repair complications caused by the first unnecessary circumcision, called revision surgery. The income from revision surgery must be added to the size of the industry. Additional surgery or surgeries may be needed due to practitioner inexperience, removing too little or too much of the foreskin, scarring, and adhesions or "skin bridges" that form during the healing process.

The intactivist organization Your Whole Baby also suggests that when a boy's foreskin is cut loose rather than high and tight, the child's penis might look as if it were not circumcised. "Upon encountering a child who has been more loosely circumcised, a doctor may pressure the family to 'revise' something that requires no revision whatsoever."[299] Thus, some revision surgeries may be as unnecessary as the first circumcision sur-

---

297 Lehman BA. The Age Old Question of Circumcision. *Boston Globe (Boston, MA)*. 1987-06-22; pp. 41+43. <cirp.org/news/bostonglobe06-22-87>.
298 AAP Speaking Points (available from the author).
299 My Child Needs to be Re-Circumcised? *Your Whole Baby.* <yourwholebaby.org/recircumcision>.

gery. If the physician knows that a boy does not need revision surgery, the recommendation to circumcise him again is yet another unfair and deceptive and fraudulent practice.

Also undisclosed and therefore unknown to parents and to the American public is that some hospitals sell the unlawfully harvested foreskins to pharmaceutical and cosmetics companies. According to the pediatrician Paul M. Fleiss in "What Your Doctor May Not Tell You About: Circumcision," a single baby foreskin contains enough genetic material to grow over 23,000 square metres of skin – or hundreds of thousands of dollars' worth of fibroblasts."[300] Because pharmaceutical companies only deal in billions of dollars, it is reasonable to suppose that the sale of foreskins produces billions more dollars of income per year for the circumcision industry, broadly defined. It would be important to learn exactly how large the revenues and profits are that pharmaceutical and cosmetics companies derive from this unlawful purchase and reuse of foreskins stolen from healthy boys' bodies.

Since circumcision is unlawful, it is unlawful for these companies to buy and resell them. Moreover, it is a federal crime under 18 U.S.C. § 2315, a crime in Massachusetts under G.L. c. 266, § 60, and likely a crime in every U.S. state, to knowingly receive, store, sell, or dispose of stolen property. Thus, once these pharmaceutical and cosmetic companies are informed that circumcision is a crime, and that the foreskins they are using are stolen property, it appears that they can be held criminally liable too.

Physicians, hospitals, American medical associations, and these pharmaceutical and cosmetics companies therefore have a multibillion dollar per year undisclosed incentive to perpetuate circumcision. That brought to mind a conversation I had with an investor, a college friend with an MBA, when I started my ecommerce business in 1999. I proposed keeping my partnership in a law firm, and he said that that would not work. Your competitors are going to be working all day every day to build their businesses, and you will need to devote 100% of your time to it. The

---

300 Quotation from VICE.com: Beauty Industry Part of Foreskin Flesh Trade, Anti-Circumcision Activists Warn. 2018-03-27. <vice.com/en/article/43bxgm/the-beauty-industry-is-part-of-a-baby-foreskin-flesh-trade-anti-circumcision-activists-warn>.

American medical profession did not build the circumcision industry by chance, but by working hard every day to sell it and to protect these multibillion dollar per year revenues from attack by opponents.

Indeed, the American Academy of Pediatrics "Task Force on Circumcision" seems to have been designed to defend the practice. The American public and parents are unlikely to know that this committee, which claims to be scientific and neutral, and which advises its member physicians to give parents neutral information about circumcision, "is not a dispassionate scientific research body: it is a medical association but also a trade association for pediatricians."[301] Thus, the AAP and that committee had a huge undisclosed financial bias in favor of preserving the income stream from male genital cutting.[1] In fact, according to Robert Van Howe, the committee consisted of a Who's Who of circumcision enthusiasts, and as discussed below, some religious adherents. It was inevitable that such a committee produced partisan guidelines.

Doctors Opposing Circumcision observed in its critique of the AAP's 2012 circumcision guidelines[302] that one committee member was a member of the AAP's finance committee, showing that the AAP was concerned about the income of its member pediatricians. The guidelines refer to member physicians as "stakeholders," a term usually reserved for investors in a for-profit enterprise.[303] Insofar as a physician's duty is to provide competent medical care that patients need, without regard to the physician's own financial interests, it is repugnant that the AAP considers physicians to be stakeholders in the business of cutting off part of healthy boys' penises.

Medical guidelines usually only contain guidance about best medical practices, but the AAP's 2012 guidelines contain an unprecedented plea

---

301 Earp BD. The AAP Report on Circumcision: Bad Science + Bad Ethics = Bad Medicine. *The Creativity Post*. 2012-09-02.
<creativitypost.com/article/the_aap_report_on_circumcision_bad_science_bad_ethics_bad_me dicine>.
302 Doctors Opposing Circumcision. Commentary on American Academy of Pediatrics 2012 Circumcision Policy Statement. 2013-04.
<doctorsopposingcircumcision.org/wp-content/uploads/2016/08/commentary-on-american-academy-of-pediatrics-2012-circumcision-policy-statement.pdf>.
303 Mehlman MJ. Why Physicians are Fiduciaries for Their Patients. *Ind Health L Rev*. 2015;12(1):8. <doi.org/10.18060/18959>

for the revival of declining Medicaid coverage. As shown in a 2011 law review article, it is unlawful to use Medicaid to pay for unnecessary genital surgery,[303] but the AAP never responded to the article (just as it never responded to the accusation that its 1989 and 1999 guidelines were fraudulent, or to the German case holding that it is a crime to circumcise boys for religious or other non-medical reasons). This shows that the committee was very concerned about the decline in Medicaid revenues. This negatively impacted the income of AAP members since Medicaid paid for about one-third of all circumcisions in 1995,[304] and likely the percentage remains similar today. The AAP is not very effective in trying to hide its overtly pro-circumcision agenda or how eager it is to revive flagging sales, revenues, and profits.

Dr. Andrew Freedman, a member of the AAP's 2012 committee, wrote in 2016 that, given the serious efforts in both the United States and Europe to ban circumcision outright, the AAP wanted to protect the option for parents to elect circumcision.[71] Protecting the option for parents to elect circumcision also conveniently protects physicians' and hospitals' profits from the practice as well as religious circumcisions.[302]

Doctors Opposing Circumcision concluded in its critique that circumcision is a "golden goose" for physicians, and that the AAP is in the business for the money of its member pediatricians.[302] Obstetricians also perform circumcisions, in fact more than pediatricians, and the American College of Obstetricians and Gynecologists (ACOG) endorsed the AAP's 2012 statement. Thus, the AAP and ACOG are both apologists for the circumcision industry, just as The Tobacco Institute, Inc. was an apologist for the U.S. tobacco industry. It put out good news about smoking while not disclosing that it is bad for health, and portrayed smoking as a personal choice. The AAP and ACOG similarly put out good news about circumcision while not disclosing that it is bad for health, and they portray it as a parental choice. Since the AAP can be sued for having issued negligent and possibly fraudulent circumcision guidelines in 2012, and ACOG endorsed the AAP's statement, ACOG can be sued on those grounds as well.[302]

---

304 Clark SJ, et al. Coverage of Newborn and Adult Male Circumcision Varies Among Public and Private US Payers Despite Health Benefits. *Health Affairs.* 2011;30:2355-6.

Professor Leonard Glick, who is Jewish, observed that Jewish American physicians were and continue to be especially vocal and influential champions of the practice, not surprisingly as most Jews believe that circumcision is commanded by their deity.[305] They have a powerful undisclosed *religious incentive* to perpetuate what is to them a sacred ritual.[302]

Undisclosed to the public, several members of the AAP's 2012 committee are believed to be Jewish. The chair of the AAP's 2012 Task Force on Circumcision was married by a rabbi.[302] Dr. Andrew Freedman stated in an interview in *The Times of Israel,* "I circumcised [my son] myself on my parents' kitchen table on the eight day of his life. But I did it for religious, not medical reasons. I did it because I had 3,000 years of ancestors looking over my shoulder."[306,307] Thus, Dr. Freedman himself stated that he made his son's penis look different not because he believed that circumcision is good for his son's health, but because of his own religious beliefs.

Petrina Fadel, who wrote a pointed critique of the AAP's 2012 guidelines,[308] recounts, "Before the AAP wrote their 2012 statement, I wrote to them and challenged them on the makeup of their Task Force. They wrote back and said there would be no religious bias in their statement." But "[t]heir 2012 statement when it came out proved otherwise to me." The guidelines assert as the AAP has long claimed that parents have the right to elect circumcision for religious reasons.[309]

---

305 Religious advocates have a religious bias in favor of circumcision and are fierce in their defense of it. See, e.g.: Darby RJL. Parental Authority, Circumcision and the Child's Right to an Open Future: Will the Real Dena Davis Please Stand Up? *Academia.edu.* 2014-09;1, 67-8. <academia.edu/8658553>.

306 Frisch M, Earp BD. Circumcision of male infants and children as a public health measure in developed countries: A critical assessment of recent evidence. *Glob Public Health.* 2018-05;13(5):626-41. <pubmed.ncbi.nlm.nih.gov/27194404>.

307 Freedman AL. Circumcision Debate: Beyond Benefits and Risks. See note #71. Dr. Freedman has also observed that most boys are circumcised because of the parents' religious, cultural, and personal preferences, which he urged is as it should be. This appears to show religious bias.

308 Fadel P. Letter to Members of the American Academy of Pediatrics' Task Force on Circumcision. 2012-08. <peacefulbeginningsrosemary.wordpress.com/circ-information/letters-to-aap>.

309 Fadel P. Email to the author. 2021-08-18.

In fact, Dr. Freedman wrote in a 2016 article that parents largely make their sons' penises look different not for medical reasons but for religious, cultural, aesthetic, familial, and personal reasons.[71] Thus, he made his son's penis look different because of his own religious and cultural beliefs. Freedman also argued in favor of a world "in which not all penises have to look the same," without providing any reason, let alone a medical reason, as one would expect from someone licensed to practice medicine, why that should be the case. Dr. Freedman appears to me to have a manifestly sincerely held but strong bias in favor of perpetuating circumcision for religious reasons having nothing to do with medicine. As mentioned, the AAP 2012 committee included a Who's Who of circumcision advocates, according to Robert Van Howe, several of whom were Jewish, likely none of whom had a foreskin, and no opponents of circumcision. The committee thus was not neutral, and it was preordained that the AAP would issue guidelines that would try to perpetuate circumcision as an industry and as a religious rite.

CULTURAL

Since physicians in the U.S. have been circumcising boys for 150 years, the practice has long been a deeply embedded cultural norm here. Physicians in the U.S. have a strong cultural bias in favor of it. Indeed, Frisch et al. wrote that it appeared obvious that the 2012 guidelines of the American Academy of Pediatrics were culturally biased.[6] In response, the AAP asserted that Europeans are biased against circumcision. That led the Yale and Oxford ethicist Brian Earp to reply:

> But let us go along with the AAP and consider their argument a bit more. Let us even concede that the mainly European authors of the 'Cultural Bias' commentary are, themselves, biased – only against circumcision rather than for it. Well … of course they are! Being biased against unnecessary surgeries performed on nonconsenting patients should be the default position of any healthcare professional worthy of the title. Such a position follows naturally from the principles of biomedical ethics that

doctors become obliged to uphold upon receiving their medical degrees. The doctors' country of origin should be of no consequence.

Let me summarize. By suggesting that a cultural norm favoring the non-therapeutic, non-consensual surgical modification of a child's penis is somehow on par with, or just as reasonable as, a medical-ethical norm favoring the avoidance of such surgery unless it is absolutely required, the AAP committee simply reveals its cultural hand.

The 'European' commentators, by contrast: 'have a clear bias against circumcision the same way they have a clear bias against parentally-elective infant toe amputation.' They should be biased against needless surgical risk, especially when the patient cannot consent. They don't even need a special 'Task Force on Leaving Boys' Genitals Alone' to prove it.

I will close with an honest suggestion. Perhaps the next time the AAP convenes a committee to consider the prudence of cutting off people's foreskins, they should think about appointing at least one member who actually has one.[301]

PERSONAL

The primary determinant of whether parents will elect to have their son circumcised or not is whether the father is circumcised. A high percentage of males in the U.S. are circumcised. Many circumcised male physicians have an unconscious but personal bias in favor of circumcision. Female physicians who have circumcised husbands and sons might also have a personal bias.

CHAPTER SUMMARY

- Physicians, hospitals, and American medical associations have undisclosed conflicts of interest and biases or motives to perpetuate circumcision.

- There is huge financial bias as circumcision is a multibillion dollar per year industry. Revenues come from neonatal circumcisions; circumcisions later in childhood; revision surgeries; the sale by hospitals of foreskins to the pharmaceutical and cosmetics industries; and the resale of the products made using them.
- There is religious bias among religious adherents.
- Physicians in the U.S. and their trade associations are culturally biased in favor of the practice, as medical experts from Europe showed.
- There may be unconscious personal bias when the physician is a circumcised male.
- Given these multiple powerful biases, it is not surprising that the American medical profession is highly motivated to perpetuate circumcision.

The question thus arises, as posed in Chapter 2 ("The Debate", Thesis, and Audience), whether the American Academy of Pediatrics and physicians who circumcise intentionally deceive parents, boys and men, and the American public about the practice. This calls for a definition of fraud.

Fraud is commonly understood to mean "trickery," "deception," or "deceit."[310] A federal Court of Appeals defined "intentional fraud" as consisting of "deception *intentionally* practiced to induce another to part with property or to surrender some legal right, and which accomplishes the end designed" (emphasis in original).[310,311] It involves a person deliberately deceiving another into *giving up something of value or something that he or she has the right to keep,* including a legal right.

There are several types of intentional fraud. There is *intentionally fraudulent conduct.* One example would be buying and selling a stock using insider information in violation of the anti-fraud provision of the Securities Exchange Act.[312,313] More commonly, intentional fraud usually consists of *false claims or misrepresentations,* but it can also include omissions, the failure to disclose what one knows and has a duty to reveal. For example, it would be a fraud to sell one's house, knowing that its foundation is being eaten away by termites, without disclosing that fact to the buyer. As discussed, a physician has a duty to disclose to the patient or proxy whatever information is material to the latter's decision.[211] It is harder to detect what physicians fail to disclose about the practice than what they do disclose.

The elements of a legal claim or "cause of action" in a lawsuit are the points that a plaintiff must prove to win the case. The elements of intentionally fraudulent representations and omissions are well established

310 Brown v. State, 868 N.E.2d 464, 466 n.1, 468 (Ind: S. Ct. 2007).
  <scholar.google.com/scholar_case?case=13501006317106502901>.
311 Bender v. Southland Corp., 749 F.2d 1205, 1216 (6th Cir. 1984).
  <scholar.google.com/scholar_case?case=5636907014620549604>.
312 Vess v. Ciba-Geigy Corp. USA, 317 F.3d 1097, 1103–04 (9th Cir. 2003).
  <scholar.google.com/scholar_case?case=665955328795694092>.
313 Kearns v. Ford Motor Co., 567 F.3d 1120 (Ct. App. 9th Cir. 2009).
  <scholar.google.com/scholar_case?case=8570538644148713283>.

under U.S. case law and are likely the same in every U.S. state. They include: "(a) misrepresentation (false representation, concealment, or nondisclosure); (b) knowledge of falsity; (c) intent to defraud, i.e., to induce reliance; (d) justifiable reliance; and (e) resulting damage."[314] Intentional fraud involves bad faith,[315] or a nefarious motive or intent to injure,[316] which can lead to an award of punitive damages.[316]

A plaintiff in a lawsuit must prove intent to defraud by clear and convincing evidence.[317] It can be difficult to prove what someone is thinking, however, so the requisite knowledge and intent to defraud may be shown by circumstantial evidence.[318]

Importantly, a plaintiff in a fraud case can also prevail on the intentional fraud claim by showing that the defendant made a representation that deceived the plaintiff with *reckless indifference as to its truth.*[319,320] Of course, physicians have a duty to be knowledgeable about medicine and they are not allowed to be recklessly indifferent to the truth in matters involving their patients.

CHAPTER SUMMARY

- Intentional fraud consists of trickery that deprives a person of something of value or of a legal right.
- Intentional fraud can include fraudulent conduct.
- The elements of fraudulent misrepresentations are:
  (a) a false claim or omission;
  (b) knowledge of its falsity;

---

314 Buckland v. Threshold Enterprises, 155 Cal. App. 4th 798, 806–07 (2007). <scholar.google.com/scholar_case?case=355169896467135107>.
315 Ryan Operations GP v. Santiam-Midwest Lumber Co., 81 F.3d 355, 361 (Ct. App, 3d. Cir. 1996). <scholar.google.com/scholar_case?case=265536197364270171>.
316 Owens-Illinois, Inc. v. Zenobia, 601 A.2d 633 (Md: Ct. App. 1992). <scholar.google.com/scholar_case?case=17610537685050847277>.
317 Larson Mfg. Co. of S.D. v. Aluminart Prod's. Ltd., 559 F.3d 1317, 1340 (Fed. Cir. 2009). <scholar.google.com/scholar_case?case=12871431717615245646>.
318 Metge v. Baehler, 762 F. 2d 621, 625 (Ct. App. 8th Cir. 1985). <scholar.google.com/scholar_case?case=16430962644382362685>.
319 Ellerin v. Fairfax Savings, 337 Md. 216 (MD: Ct. App. 1995). <scholar.google.com/scholar_case?case=10648071527486395508>.
320 Fraudulent Misrepresentation. *Legal Information Inst.* <law.cornell.edu/wex/fraudulent_misrepresentation>.

(c) intent to defraud;

(d) justifiable reliance; and

(e) resulting damage.

- Circumstantial evidence can be used to prove intent to defraud.
- A defendant can also be held liable for intentional fraud for making a false claim or omission with reckless indifference as to its truth.

17   FRAUDULENT ADVERTISING AND MARKETING

Some hospitals and medical practices promote circumcision in their websites and other marketing materials by making false claims and by not telling readers the truth about the procedure.

As a notable example, in 2012, the American Academy of Pediatrics sent its members confidential "Circumcision Speaking Points" to help them answer questions that the media might pose in response to the AAP's widely publicized pro-circumcision guidelines.[321] The Speaking Points are all biased in favor of circumcision. As examples, the AAP claimed that it revised its 1999 policy statement because new studies shows that circumcision has more medical benefits than previously known including prevention of HIV. But the AAP knows that circumcision does not prevent HIV: the real claim is that at best it slightly reduces the risk of contracting it. The AAP cannot prove its offhanded claim that pain "is easily addressed." The AAP asks, if the primary medical benefits (which are actually unproven potential medical benefits) involve the prevention of sexually transmitted diseases, why circumcise newborns? The best answer the AAP was able to produce is that some adolescents have sexual intercourse, hardly a compelling reason to circumcise newborn boys. The AAP falsely claims, "Many of the medical society statements that have been characterized as opposing newborn circumcision do not really oppose newborn circumcision." For example, the Royal Dutch Medical Association condemns the practice. In answer to the question, "Why does the AAP support male circumcision but oppose female genital cutting?," it answered,

> The two procedures are not analogous. Female genital cutting is mutilation. Female genital cutting is not circumcision. The scientific evidence of female genital cutting indicates only harms and no health benefits. In male circumcision, the anatomy is different, and the procedure is different. Male circumcision has been shown scientifically to provide benefits to the

---

321 Available from the author.

person being circumcised and has a proven track record for safety.[321]

This answer is disingenuous as the anatomy and physiology of the prepuce is very similar in the male and the female. It is risky, harmful, unethical, and unlawful to amputate the prepuce regardless of gender. The American Academy of Pediatrics states in its Speaking Points that a circumcision can cost upwards of $1,750, and claims that insurance should cover it, and that the AAP is taking this stance because the issue is about "health care," not profits. Cutting off a healthy part of a person's body without his or her consent is not "health care," however, and physicians are not allowed to perform or to pay themselves for performing unnecessary surgery on a child. The claims in the Speaking Points are not neutral at all but rather are designed, like the guidelines they defend, to sell circumcision for the financial benefits of physicians and hospitals, and to give physicians cover when asked about it by the media and parents.

As another example of misleading marketing, a hospital in New Hampshire markets circumcision with a colorful picture of happy boys and girls with balloons, as if being circumcised is like having a wonderful day playing games in a park. The hospital claims that "Circumcision of your newborn son is recommended by the American Academy of Pediatrics,"[322] a patently false claim because no national medical association in the United States has ever recommended it. The hospital also lists as benefits easier genital hygiene, when there is soap; and, as always, "[s]ocial/cultural/religious reasons, which might benefit parents but not their sons."

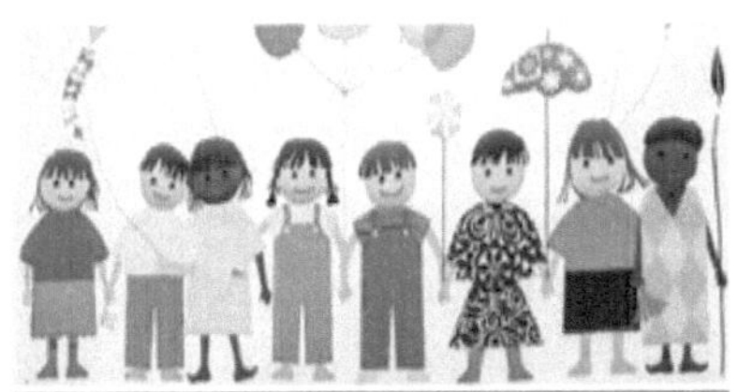
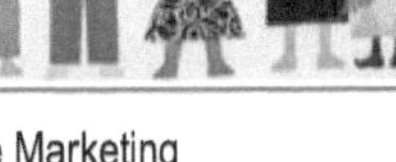
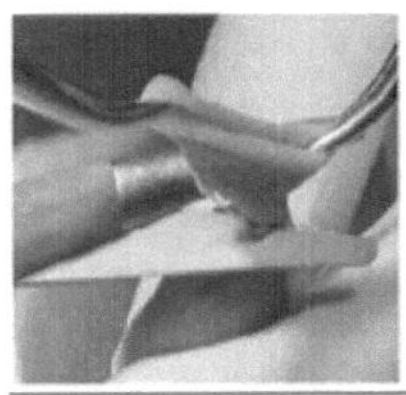
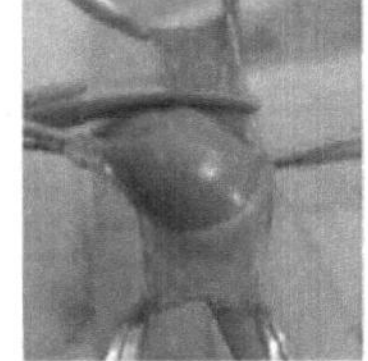

The Marketing   The Reality

322 Pediatrics Circumcision Information. *Monadnock Community Hospital.*
    <monadnockcommunityhospital.com/services/pediatrics/circumcision-information>.

The website for Harvard University's Children's Hospital in Boston likewise suggests that it is easier for parents and ultimately the child to clean the circumcised penis, even though the hospital goes on to acknowledge that boys can learn to wash the penis using soap and water around the time of toilet training.[323] It is safe to say that the hospital does not offer other surgeries as preventative measures in lieu of hygiene. The hospital also calls circumcision a "deeply personal choice" for parents, which will require consideration of religious, cultural, and personal as well as medical factors.[323] It is a deeply personal choice, but for circumcised boys and men to make, not their parents. It is safe to say that the hospital does not offer invite parents to elect to have other surgeries performed on their child for reasons having nothing to do with medicine. Children's Hospital calls circumcision common in the U.S., which fails to disclose that it is uncommon outside the United States except for religious reasons. The hospital's website also asserts that "Once the procedure is completed the child will not have pain with urination …" This fails to disclose that circumcised boys experience post-operative pain. Neither of these hospitals discloses that the foreskin is highly erogenous and the most sensitive part of the penis, which every parent needs to know.

In its circumcision marketing materials, ThedaCare, a health care provider in the Northeast and Wisconsin, does not disclose anything about the foreskin that circumcision removes. It claims, "The healthcare provider will gently loosen the foreskin from around the head of the penis, making a small slit in the foreskin." Gently loosen the foreskin? Separating the two is like removing nails from their nail bed, a form of torture. The site michigancircumcision.com similarly claims that its clinic provides "a gentle and safe method for babies,"[324] when the procedure is neither gentle nor safe for babies or older boys. It also claims that the doctor's "circumcision technique provides outstanding cosmetic results with minimal discomfort," but the boys who are circumcised and the men they become might beg to differ that the appearance of their denuded penis is outstanding or that the discomfort was minimal. The website gentlecircumcision.com also pitches its services as "Gentle Circumcision,"

323 <childrenshospital.org/conditions-and-treatments/treatments/circumcision>.
324 <michigancircumcision.com>.

and depicts a happy boy grateful to have been circumcised. Many boys are not happy or grateful but rather enraged that they were. Kaiser Permanente's website falsely claims, "If your baby is a boy, you and your partner must decide whether to circumcise him." Parents do not need to make that decision. Moreover, Kaiser Permanente should have stated, "decide whether to circumcise him or not."

In short, these marketing materials, found at random – likely there are many other examples – contain clearly false and thus apparently intentional false and fraudulent claims. They promote circumcision to unsuspecting parents without telling the truth about it.

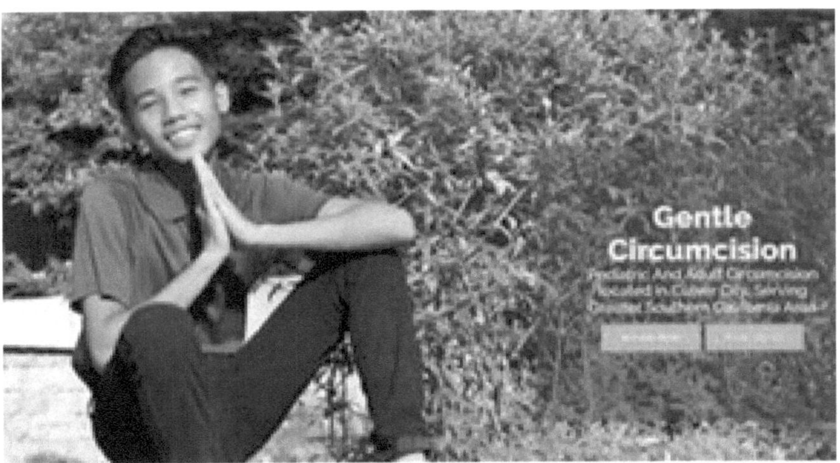

If circumcision were as gentle and beneficial as the American medical profession portrays it, men would choose it for themselves.

CHAPTER SUMMARY

- Physicians, hospitals, and American medical associations use false and fraudulent advertising and marketing to pre-sell circumcision to expectant parents, and in an attempt to justify it to the American public.
- Examples include portraying circumcision as a walk in a park, as gentle, as safe, and as cleaner, with outstanding cosmetic results, and falsely claiming that parents must decide whether to have their son circumcised or not.

18   Fraudulent Conduct in the Hospital

It is granted that most physicians and nurses work extremely hard and provide competent and compassionate care to their patients. In fact, many physicians have provided heroic medical care during the COVID-19 pandemic, at risk to their own health and lives and that of their families. It is also granted that medical students may know nothing about circumcision, and that they are taught and paid to "see one, do one, teach one."

That having been said, there is an enormous amount of unnecessary surgery. The only reason for a physician or surgeon to operate on a healthy person is for monetary gain. As Chapter 14 (The Past as Prelude to the Present) showed, physicians used unfair and deceptive practices to build the circumcision industry. The past is prelude to the present as medical professionals and their trade associations continue to engage in the same and new deceptive practices today.

Permission Hidden in Admission Forms

In the past, some hospitals used admission forms that contained permission to circumcise. Parents would not have expected this in the rush of admission to a hospital to give birth, and few parents would have noticed this provision. Parents who do not speak English would not have been able to read the admission form even if they tried to do so. To the extent that hospitals continue to engage in this practice today, it constitutes fraudulent conduct.

Targeting Infants Unable to Object

The historian Robert Darby explains how physicians target infants and other young boys unable to object:

> By the turn of the century, it was accepted that circumcision was generally desirable as a means of preventing masturbation, phimosis, venereal disease, certain forms of cancer, and various minor penis problems ... as well as reducing the male sex drive

(Darby, 2005). Most of the real medical problems in this list occurred in adults rather than children, but because *adult men were not exhibiting much eagerness to get themselves circumcised,* the doctors concentrated on the younger generation. As David Gollaher (2000) summed up, 'The ultimate popularity of circumcision depended not on convincing normal men to undergo the ordeal of surgery, but on *targeting a group of patients who could not object'* (emphasis added).[325]

TARGETING OLDER BOYS AND IGNORING THEIR PREFERENCES

Part of the sales pitch for circumcising newborn boys is the claim that circumcision is best performed in infancy, as the physician told me. The claim is that the risk of complications is higher later in childhood; that older boys will need general anesthesia; and that it will cost more. (This book argues, of course, that boys should not be circumcised at any age. Ignoring that, the argument could be made that it is better to wait until boys are older. They can be asked whether they want to be circumcised or not. The foreskin may have separated from the head of the penis, so it will not be necessary to force them apart. General anesthesia can be used, as it typical for surgery. And they could ask for post-surgical pain relief.) One would expect, then, that physicians in the U.S. would not circumcise older boys, and that they would warn against it. But in the face of declining circumcision rates among newborn boys, physicians have changed their tune, and they are increasingly circumcising older boys as well.

A mother informed me, "I was solicited for circumcision when I was at my 6 weeks checkup after birth, with my young son with me. I couldn't believe he asked me that, but it was his last chance, so he had the gall to ask."

---

325 Darby RJL. Targeting Patients Who Cannot Object? Re-Examining the Case for Non-Therapeutic Infant Circumcision. *Sage Open.* 2016-06-03. <journals.sagepub.com/doi/10.1177/2158244016649219>.

When Florida stopped using Medicaid to pay for neonatal circumcisions,[326] when most circumcisions are performed, the number of circumcisions paid for by Medicaid should have gone down dramatically. Instead, according to a study, the number went up.[326] The authors of the study attribute this to medically indicated circumcisions performed later in childhood and circumcisions needed to treat persistent phimosis or a tight foreskin. The implication is that if you do not circumcise a boy at birth, it will be necessary to circumcise him later. But it is rarely necessary to circumcise any boy during childhood.[118] The foreskin usually separates naturally from the glans penis by puberty;[284] and when it does not, a tight foreskin can usually be treated by steroids and stretching.[110] Accordingly, unable to get paid to circumcise healthy boys at birth, physicians began circumcising healthy boys later in childhood, and using false diagnoses to get reimbursed such as a tight foreskin.

In addition, when older boys say that they do not want to be circumcised, physicians are required to respect their preferences. The American Academy of Pediatrics has acknowledged this:

> Patients should participate in decision-making commensurate with their development; they should provide assent to care whenever reasonable. Parents and physicians should not exclude children and adolescents from decision-making without persuasive reasons. Indeed, some patients have specific legal entitlements to either consent or to refuse medical intervention. … Only patients who have appropriate decisional capacity and legal empowerment can give their informed consent to medical care. In all other situations, parents or other surrogates provide informed permission for diagnosis and treatment of children with the assent of the child whenever appropriate.[207]

In the *Hironimus* case, however, the physician ignored the boys' preference not to be circumcised. Insofar as it can be inferred that no boy

---

326 Soto S, et al. Impact of Florida Medicaid guidelines on frequency and cost of delayed circumcision at Nemours Children's hospital. *J Ped Urol.* 2022-03-07. <jpurol.com/article/S1477-5131(22)00099-7/pdf>

wants to be circumcised, physicians should not be targeting any of these older boys.

TARGETING LEGALLY INCAPACITATED MOTHERS

Medical professionals also solicit the parents' permission one or two days after the mother has labored for hours, usually on medications, or has had a Cesarean Section, has given birth, and may be nursing her newborn son. In retrospect, when the physician asked me *The Question*, my wife was "glassy eyed" and "out of it," although I was unaware of that at the time. Thus, the mothers from whom nurses or physicians solicit consent are often legally incapacitated, and their permission is not legally valid.

It is a physician's job to determine whether a patient or the patient's proxy, here the mother, is competent to make a medical decision. Physicians make that determination on a regular basis. Using the precautionary principle of "better safe than sorry," physicians should assume that any mother who has recently given birth is legally incapacitated. They should not pitch circumcision to mothers in the hospital when they are mentally, emotionally, and physically exhausted from an event that is typically arduous, intensely painful, and performed with medications.

PROCEEDING WITH ONLY ONE PARENT'S PERMISSION, EVEN OVER THE OBJECTION OF THE OTHER

Physicians also gain an unfair advantage when they exclude one parent from the conversation, when they proceed with the circumcision when only one of the two parents has assented, and when they proceed over the objection of one of the parents, as in spite circumcision cases. The physician who solicited my permission zeroed in on me and kept his back turned to my wife. He made no effort to include her. Children have two parents, not one. In Europe, boys are rarely circumcised, but when they are, both parents must agree. The physician took unfair advantage of me by not including my wife, a physician, in the conversation, and by not waiting until she had recovered from giving birth on medications.

The U.S. ethicist Douglas Diekema wrote (before he became the main spokesperson for the AAP in 2012) that boys should not be circumcised unless both parents agree to it.[212] If parents had the right to elect circumcision, which they do not, both parents should be required to elect it, given the deleterious impact on their son's health and well-being, as well as the possibility of parental regret, which physicians do not tell parents about either. It is also unfair to circumcise a boy over one parent's objection, as happens in spite circumcision cases where the physician ignores the mother's desperate pleas.

SURPRISE

When my son was born, *The Question* took me by surprise, and it must take many other parents by surprise as well. The American Academy of Pediatrics knows, and physicians must know, that this takes unfair advantage of the parents. Susan Blank, the chair of the AAP's 2012 committee, herself said in a press release, "It's a good idea to have this conversation during pregnancy ... so you have time to make the decision."[327] She thereby acknowledged that it is a bad idea for physicians to ask this question in the hospital when the parents will not have enough time to make a fully informed decision, as commonly happens. Moreover, adults sometimes obtain a second opinion before consenting to surgery. Parents solicited in the hospital will not have that option.[327] This is analogous to the obstetric violence that is common in Brazil, where many physicians advance specious reasons to perform Cesarean sections and episiotomies, which pay better than normal childbirth, using false diagnoses as ridiculous as "hairy baby." A New York Times reporter who gave birth in Brazil writes,

> In Brazilian private facilities, C-section rates are even higher than in public hospitals, reaching 84.6 percent. The procedure is more profitable for these institutions, which must think about

327 New Evidence Points to Greater Benefits of Infant Circumcision, But Final Say is Still Up to Parents, Says AAP. <web.archive.org/web/20120830054327/http://www.aap.org/en-us/about-the-aap/aap-press-room/pages/New-Benefits-Point-to-Greater-Benefits-of-Infant-Circumcision-But-Final-Say-is-Still-Up-to-parents-Says-AAP.aspx>

money, and more convenient for doctors, who don't have to wait hours for the natural processes of labor to unfold. And so, C-sections are routinely prescribed *under an endless number of pretexts,* many of them as implausible as: placental allergies, asthma, scoliosis, gingivitis, an excessively hairy baby, a soccer match between Atlético and Cruzeiro, and – most creative of all – the assumption that evolution made the female body incompatible with labor. – Surgery is the rule; vaginal childbirth is the exception. So when I expressed my desire to let nature take its course ahead of the birth of my daughter two months ago, my ob-gyn told me she would assent 'only if everything goes perfectly until the due date.' She didn't seem to notice that her logic was inverted – natural labor should be the default unless something goes wrong – but perhaps that was to be expected from a physician who, according to insurance records, has an 80 percent C-section rate (emphasis added).[328]

Circumcision in the U.S. is just like childbirth in Brazil. There is never a need to circumcise a newborn boy, and it is rarely necessary to circumcise an older boy, but any excuse for it will do. And if any excuse fails to convince, physicians try another one.

Fathers, who may be left to make the circumcision decision on their own, also may be tired, distracted, and caught off guard, as I was, and unable to think clearly. In addition, nurses and physicians give the parents only a few minutes to decide the permanent fate of their son's foreskin. This constitutes unlawful undue influence and duress or pressure, which invalidates the parental permission.[328]

RELENTLESS SOLICITATIONS AND BADGERING

Doctors sometimes claim that they circumcise baby boys because the parents ask that they be circumcised, and no doubt some parents do ask.

328 Barbara V. Hairy Baby? Better Get a C-section. Gingivitis? C-section. Scoliosis? C-section. *NY Times.* 2018-08-27. "C-sections are routinely prescribed under an endless number of pretexts, many of them … implausible." <nytimes.com/2018/08/27/opinion/cesarean-section-childbirth-brazil.html>.

In talking with many mothers, however, nurses or physicians offered it to them – they did not ask – and mothers do not ask in Europe. A survey in January 2021 by the charitable organization Intact America shows for the most part physicians create the demand for circumcision. The survey defined "solicitation" as every time a physician, midwife, or nurse either verbally asked the mother whether she wanted to have her son circumcised; recommended that she circumcise her son; told her (falsely) that circumcision is required; handed her a circumcision consent form; or assumed (without verifying it) that the mother wanted her son circumcised. The survey results revealed:

- Physicians or nurses solicited 94% of mothers to have their baby boys circumcised.
- 78% of mothers solicited agreed to have their sons circumcised.
- "Soft sells," such as being handed a consent form, increased circumcisions by 137%.
- The average number of solicitations was eight.
- Solicitation, in all forms, increased circumcisions by 173%.
- Physicians were responsible for three out of 5 solicitations; nurses and midwives were responsible for the remainder.
- The mothers were also told that private insurance or the government would pay for it 84% of the time, another incentive to elect it.

The pediatrician Robert Van Howe informed me years ago that it is common in Michigan for physicians to badger the parents like this. As an example of this, Steven Svoboda, founder of Attorneys for the Rights of the Child reports that when his son was born, nurses asked him and his wife *The Question* on five separate occasions, even though they had said "no" at the outset and continued to refuse the procedure every time that nurses proposed it.[329] Svoboda finally became exasperated and told the last nurse, "You know, there is no medical need for this," which the nurse should have been telling him and his wife to begin with because parents may not know that. While writing this book, another mother informed me:

---

329 Personal communication from J. Steven Svoboda.

> I talked to the female doctor in charge [at Highland Hospital in
> Rochester] and said how my daughter had been badgered
> 8 times to circumcise her son. She had to tell them NO 8 times!
> I said that this should never happen to anyone, and that all the
> nurses had to do was look at her chart and see that she had said
> NO to circumcision in her birth plan. Even if she was asked
> once [and said no once], that should have been written down in
> her chart, and that should have been the end of it.[330]

In short, in many hospitals in the United States, nurses and physicians, who have more authority, aggressively solicit permission, refuse to take "no" for an answer, even a "no" written in a chart (which in my experience medical professionals regularly check and follow). They also solicit the parents' permission eight times, on *average*.[331] Medical professionals are truly relentless in trying to sell circumcision! They refuse to take "no" for an answer.

A reviewer asked me whether the study commissioned by Intact America was peer reviewed. It does not matter. Physicians bear the burden of justifying circumcision and, assuming that they could do that, of obtaining fully informed and freely given parental permission for it. Now that the opponents of circumcision have made a credible claim that physicians solicit and badger parents on average eight times, the burden falls on physicians to rebut the accusation, and to prove that they do not badger parents.

Physicians and nurses must know that badgering is unfair to parents and thereby to their sons. It constitutes a clear breach of fiduciary duty or trust. It also constitutes undue influence, defined as "influence by which a person is induced to act otherwise than by their own free will or without adequate attention to the consequences."[332] The nurses must be acting under orders from the hospital and/or the attending physician to do so. By

---

330 Private conversation.

331 Ashford J. Having a Baby Boy? Intact America Having a Baby Boy? Intact America Warns, "Get Ready for the Circumcision Sellers!". *NY Times.* 2020;18.
<prweb.com/releases/having_a_baby_boy_intact_america_warns_get_ready_for_the_circumci sion_sellers/prweb17552844.htm>.

332 Definition of "undue influence." <google.com/search?q=undue%2Binfluence>.

contrast, as Svoboda observed during a radio interview, when parents say "yes" at the outset in response to *The Question,* nurses do not ask them again once, let alone many times, whether they want to learn more about circumcision or whether they might want to get a second opinion or change their minds.

Once parents say "yes," the son is whisked away and his foreskin is cut off at the first opportunity, before the parents can change their mind. The Jewish rabbi Maimonides stated that if left uncircumcised for years, the parents' love for their child would grow and they would not elect to have him circumcised. The boy in turn might not choose it for himself.[39] Medical professionals know that if parents leave the hospital with their son's penis intact, they are not coming back to have him circumcised.

Badgering also constitutes duress, defined as any action brought to bear on someone to do something against their will or better judgment,[333] and as exerting pressure upon another to induce him to act in a manner that he or she otherwise would not have.[334] A philosopher defines coercion as, "the practice of compelling a person or manipulating them to behave in an involuntary way (whether through action or inaction) by use of threats, intimidation, trickery, or some other form of pressure or force. These are used as leverage, to force the victim to act in the desired way." Badgering is another unfair and deceptive and fraudulent tactic.

In an often-cited case, *Canterbury v. Spence,* the court stated that it is "clear that the consent, to be efficacious, must be free from imposition upon the patient [or proxy]. It is the settled rule that therapy not authorized by the patient may amount to a tort – a common law battery – by the physician."[335] Permission obtained by surprise, by high pressure sales tactics, by badgering, and by coercion is legally invalid, giving boys, men, and their parents claims against the physician and hospital for battery or an unlawful touching and for breach of fiduciary duty or trust.

---

333 Definition of "duress." <google.com/search?q=duress>.
334 Black's Law dictionary (6th ed.) defines "duress" as, "any ... coercion used... to induce another to act [or not act] in a manner [they] otherwise would not [or would]."
335 Canterbury v. Spence, 464 F.2d 772, 782–83 (D.C. Cir. 1972).

- Physicians and nurses engage in fraudulent conduct in the hospital.
- They target infants and older boys unable to object.
- They target legally incapacitated mothers, whose permission is legally invalid.
- They give parents only minutes to decide, a high-pressure sales tactic and unlawful duress.
- Physicians or nurses solicit parental permission eight times on average.
- When parents say "no," physicians and nurses often badger them until they relent, which constitutes duress and undue influence.
- Hospitals may hide permission to circumcise in their admission forms, as in the past.
- Medical professionals can be relentless in pressuring parents to elect to have their son circumcised.

As in the past (Chapter 14, The Past as Prelude to the Present), medical professionals continue to advance frivolous or specious, which is to say just plain dumb, and thus plainly indefensible and fraudulent reasons to circumcise boys and to persuade parents to elect it.

For example, in 2012, the American Academy of Pediatrics stated that circumcision is one of the most common procedures in the world.[336] Drilling holes in the brain to release evil spirits was common once too.

The AAP cited a study showing that moisture on the glans is more common in "uncircumcised men" and a marker of poor penile hygiene.[337] Essentially the AAP is claiming, as has been common throughout history, that the foreskin is dirty or bad for health. In fact, it is good for health that the foreskin is a moist mucous membrane, as this facilitates comfortable manipulation and sexual intercourse.

The AAP stated that "[m]ale circumcision performed during the newborn period has considerably lower complication rates than when performed later in life." This is a frivolous argument, as it is unnecessary to expose boys to any risk of complications at any time during childhood. Moreover, by the time boys reach puberty, the foreskin of their penis will have separated from the glans, so it will not need to be pried apart; general anesthetic can be used to prevent pain during the operation; and the boys will be able to request post-operative pain relief.

The AAP stated, "Newborn males who are not circumcised at birth are much less likely to elect circumcision in adolescence or early adulthood."[338] Newborn boys do not elect circumcision – it is forced upon them – and adolescent boys and men rarely elect it either.

The AAP stated in 2012, "Parents are entitled to factually correct, nonbiased information about circumcision and should receive this information from clinicians before conception or early in pregnancy, which is

336 2012 AAP Technical Report (Abstract).
    <pediatrics.aappublications.org/content/pediatrics/130/3/e756.pdf>.
337 2012 AAP Technical Report at e763.
    <pediatrics.aappublications.org/content/pediatrics/130/3/e756.pdf>.
338 2012 AAP Technical Report at e760.
    <pediatrics.aappublications.org/content/pediatrics/130/3/e756.pdf>.

when parents typically make circumcision decisions." Parents are entitled to neutral and unbiased information, but they will not get it from the AAP. Parents also typically make the circumcision decision in the hospital and not before.

In a 2016 article,[339] Douglas Diekema of the 2012 American Academy of Pediatrics committee on circumcision and colleagues wrote: "All evidence-based policy statements support [infant male circumcision] on medical grounds. Thus [it] is not, 'unnecessary surgery'." Of course, it is unnecessary surgery! National policy statements opposed to circumcision cite scientific evidence too; they just reach the opposite conclusion that healthy boys should not be circumcised. The authors of the article then complain that opponents call circumcision an "amputation": "that term is inaccurate and reflects emotive anti-circumcision rhetoric."[339] That term is accurate, however, as to "amputate" is "to remove by cutting."[340] Moreover, an article in American Family Physician itself states that all methods of circumcision conclude with "amputation of the foreskin."[341] The authors of the 2016 article falsely claim that circumcision does not destroy the mobility of the penis,[339] when it is self-evident that removing the foreskin prevents it from moving back and forth as the anatomically correct penis can do.

The American Academy of Pediatrics claims in the 2016 article that parents should consider social reasons, and that parents are motivated by social concerns (such as having a father or brother who was circumcised).[342] Social concerns and the desire to conform to a social norm are specious reasons that physicians could advance to justify female genital cutting, scarification, or any other harmful bodily modification.

The AAP also stated that circumcision has a protective effect against cervical cancer. No one would promote female genital cutting with the

339 Diekema DS, et al. Critical Evaluation of Adler's Challenge to the CDC's Male Circumcision Recommendations. *Int J Children's Rights.* 2016-07;24(2):265-303. <researchgate.net/publication/305695358>.
340 Merriam Webster dictionary, definition of "amputate." <merriam-webster.com/dictionary/amputate>.
341 Rose V. AAP Updates Its Recommendations on Circumcision. *Am Fam Physician.* 1999-05-15;59(10):2918-9. <aafp.org/afp/1999/0515/p2918.html>.
342 2012 AAP Technical Report at e762. <pediatrics.aappublications.org/content/pediatrics/130/3/e756.pdf>.

argument that it might reduce cancer or another disease in a male. There is no legal duty to cut off part of one's body on the off chance that it might benefit some as yet unknown person in the future.

A 2002 study claims that the conventional sleeve technique "produces a satisfactory cosmetic result."[343] According to whom? Increasing numbers of circumcised men are unhappy with the appearance of their surgically altered penis.

Recently a Chinese mother and a mother of Brazilian descent told me that they would not have asked to have their son circumcised. When asked, neither wanted their son to be. But in both cases, the physician gave the new mothers the frivolous arguments that the circumcised penis is cleaner, that the baby will not remember it, and that circumcision is better performed in infancy, when it is better not performed at all. The Chinese mother told the doctor, my son is only one day old, and to wait. She thus intuited that newborn boys are fragile. The physician said her son should be circumcised as soon as possible, a false claim because it is never necessary to circumcise a healthy boy. The only urgency was that if the mother left the hospital with her son genitally intact, she would never have brought him back to be circumcised. The mother signed a permission form, but she did not read it, and could not have understood it as her English was rudimentary at the time. Her son was circumcised the second day after his birth instead of the first. Both mothers said that their son was returned with his penis wrapped in a bandage with blood on it; both mothers said they felt their son's pain; and both said they regretted having given permission. The Chinese woman said she feels that she trusted the doctor but that he took unfair advantage of her and her son. The boy will no doubt be dismayed to learn when he returns to China that he is the only boy missing the foreskin of his penis.

To summarize, some medical professionals continue to this day to use the same frivolous reasons as they did in the past to sell genital cutting to unsuspecting parents.

---

343 Brisson PA, Patel HI, Feins NR. Revision of circumcision in children: Report of 56 cases. *J Pediatr Surg.* 2002-09;37(9):1346-6. <pubmed.ncbi.nlm.nih.gov/12194129/>

CHAPTER SUMMARY

- Just as in the past, physicians and their medical associations make frivolous arguments in favor of circumcision today.
- These include the arguments that the procedure is common; that boys should be circumcised at birth because they are unlikely to choose it later for themselves; that parents should consider social reasons; that the circumcised penis is cleaner; that the boy will not remember it; and that circumcision is best performed in infancy, when it is best not performed at all.

Chapter 3 showed that genital cutting is very bad for health: it seriously harms all boys and men. For example, it meets every part of the definition of "substantial bodily injury" under the Massachusetts child abuse law: "bodily injury which creates a permanent disfigurement, protracted loss or impairment of a function of a body member, limb or organ, or substantial risk of death."[344] Like female genital cutting, male genital cutting also meets the definition of "mutilation", "an act or instance of destroying, removing, or severely damaging a limb or other body part of a person." This chapter suggests that the most recent, widely publicized 2012 circumcision guidelines of the American Academy of Pediatrics hide the fact that circumcision is bad for health. Essentially, the AAP continues to falsely portray circumcision as a common, simple, safe, and harmless snip of a useless piece of skin, or nearly so. Medical professionals in turn are also unlikely to disclose the risks and harms of the operation to parents.

NOT MEDICALLY NECESSARY

As stated above, it is rarely medically necessary to circumcise any boy in childhood or a man in adulthood,[344] and it is never medically necessary to circumcise a healthy boy. The AAP's guidelines in 2012[94] and physicians should expressly disclose that to parents, who may not realize it.

NOT ROUTINE OR COMMON

Physicians who circumcise portray circumcision as routine, and it was called routine infant circumcision in the recent past, whereas no operation is routine for the person upon whom it is performed. The American Academy of Pediatrics similarly claims that circumcision "is one of the most common procedures in the world,"[345] falsely implying that it is one of the

---

344 MGL c. 265, § 13J.
345 2012 AAP Technical Report (Abstract).
   <pediatrics.aappublications.org/content/pediatrics/130/3/e756.pdf>.

most common *medical* procedures in the world. Physicians in most countries outside the United States leave the genitals of healthy boys alone,[94] and most boys are circumcised for religious reasons, not for medical reasons.

NOT A SIMPLE PROCEDURE, AND OPERATORS ARE UNLIKELY TO BE WELL TRAINED

The American medical profession calls circumcision as a "simple procedure," whether by saying that it is (as the physician told the author) or by omission (the public assumes that it is). Calling it a "procedure" makes it sound simple and benign, whereas calling it "surgery" would set off alarm bells. (Similarly, the profession describes the anatomically correct penis as "uncircumcised," as if it is defective and in need of a circumcision. Thus, the claim that it is better to be circumcised than not is embedded in the English language. Notably, physicians do not refer to anatomically correct female genitalia as uncircumcised.)

Granted, circumcision is a simple procedure compared to heart and brain surgery, but it is not simple. For example, physicians who use a clamp cannot see how much foreskin is going to be removed. In addition, in the newborn, the penis is tiny. Thus, any small error will be amplified many times over in the adult penis, especially when it is erect. For example, "high and tight" circumcisions, as are common in the United States, do not leave enough tissue to accommodate a comfortable erection, and can draw pubic hair onto the penis. The AAP knows that circumcision surgery is not simple, as it states that "[m]ale circumcision should be performed by trained and competent practitioners."[346] It knows that "untrained providers who perform circumcisions have more complications than well-trained providers who perform the procedure, regardless of whether the former are physicians, nurses, or traditional religious providers."[347] The AAP emphasizes that "it is imperative that those providing circumcision are adequately trained,"[347] and it recommends that

346 2012 AAP Technical Report, p. e757.
   <pediatrics.aappublications.org/content/pediatrics/130/3/e756.pdf>.
347 2012 AAP Technical Report, p. e756.
   <pediatrics.aappublications.org/content/pediatrics/130/3/e756.pdf>.

professional organizations including the AAP develop standards of trainee proficiency.[346] The AAP thus knows that operators are often not well trained and that it is not doing its job to develop standards so that they will be. Moreover, sometimes circumcisions are not even performed by physicians, but by nurses, midwives, and medical students. Parents are unlikely to know this or to be told.

NOT PAINLESS OR WELL TOLERATED

Medical professionals are unlikely to tell parents that circumcision is painful, even though that has been known since ancient times. The American Academy of Pediatrics acknowledged in 1999 that, "There is considerable evidence that newborns who are circumcised without analgesia experience pain and physiologic stress."[348] The technical report supporting the 2012 AAP guidelines also claims, "The procedure is well tolerated when performed by trained professionals under sterile conditions with appropriate pain management." Often those who perform the operation are not well trained, and often no anesthetic is used. The AAP knows that as it wrote, "adequate analgesia should be provided whenever newborn circumcision is performed."[346] It is difficult to imagine that a newborn boy would tolerate well having the most sensitive part of his body forced off the head of his penis, clamped under thousands of pounds of pressure, and cut off, without general anesthesia. Publicly available on-line videos of newborn boys undergoing the operation suggest that the boys are in great pain. A man who is active in the Stop the Cut Foundation, an organization opposed to forced genital cutting in Africa, writes, "I still remember and see the pain I went through. I wouldn't wish that to even my worst enemy." As noted in Chapter 4 (Is Genital Cutting Good or Bad For Health?), genital cutting was performed on enemies and young adults in order to cause them pain. And if AAP's claim were true that pain is well tolerated when local anesthetic is used, physicians would not need to use general anesthesia when circumcising older boys.

---

348 AAP Task Force on Circumcision. 1999 AAP Circumcision Policy Statement. *Pediatrics.* 1999-03-01;103(3):686-93. <cirp.org/library/statements/aap1999>.

The 2012 guidelines also fail to disclose that male genital cutting causes untreated post-operative pain, which infants are not able to report; that it can cause behavioral changes; that it may impair neurological development;[94] or that its own committee on pain urged physicians to prevent causing pain to infants whenever possible. Therefore, the AAP downplayed and did not disclose the truth about the pain that circumcision causes in 2012, just as it had failed to do from 1989 to 1999.[306] Indeed, the American medical profession has hidden and understated the pain for the past 150 years. If parents had any idea how painful the procedure is, most would decline the invitation to elect it.

NOT SAFE

When the AAP issued its widely publicized 2012 circumcision guidelines, it sent its member pediatrics confidential "Circumcision Speaking Points" intended to help AAP members prepare for media interviews. Not by chance, the speaking or talking points would also help physicians prepare for questions that the parents of newborn boys might have when offered the procedure. The Speaking Points claim that circumcision has a "proven track record of safety." Thus, the AAP expressly claims, and advises its member physicians to tell parents, that circumcision is safe when it is not. Medical professionals in turn are unlikely to tell parents that circumcision is unsafe, because if they did, the parents would not elect it, so they imply by omission that it is safe. As discussed in Chapter 4 (Is Genital Cutting Good or Bad For Health?), and as shown in Van Howe's affidavit in the appendix, circumcision can cause more than 50 different complications, so it is not safe at all.

The AAP's next false claim is that "[c]omplications are infrequent; most are minor, and severe complications are rare."[94] This intentionally downplays complications and willfully misleads parents. The AAP admitted in its Technical Report that it does not know the rate and severity of complications following the procedure, as Douglas Gairdner had observed in 1949, sixty-three years earlier.[349]

---

349 2012 AAP Technical Report, p. e772.3.
<pediatrics.aappublications.org/content/pediatrics/130/3/e756.pdf>.

The AAP also understated the complication rate. Dr. Brady of the AAP committee claimed during a debate a significant, acute complication rate of 1 in 500 infants circumcised or 0.2%. European centers report a 1.2% to 3.8% complication rate in both the newborn and non-newborn periods (between 6 and 19 times higher).[349] But clinical studies report an average post-circumcision rate of meatal stenosis alone of 5% to 20%.[350] Insofar as circumcision removes living and erogenous tissue, the true risk of an adverse outcome is 100%.

In 1999, the AAP listed some of the many minor and serious injuries that circumcision can cause, but it did not disclose them again in 2012, so it intentionally hid them in 2012. The AAP should have disclosed again in 2012 as it had done in 1999 that "badly performed circumcisions, causing discomfort or poor cosmetic outcomes, often necessitating repeat operations and repair jobs, are *common"* (emphasis added).[351]

The AAP is also hiding the fact that male genital cutting can be fatal when performed by physicians in a nonsterile hospital setting.[352] That has been known since Gairdner disclosed it in his famous paper in 1949.[83] By contrast, the Royal Australasian College of Physicians (RACP) disclosed that fact in its 2010 circumcision policy statement: "Infection is usually minor but uncommonly septicemia and meningitis may occur and rarely these complications may lead to death, even in modern times in modern health systems."[353]

Nor did the AAP disclose in 2012 that male genital cutting can cause psychological harm,[94] and that boys and men may be angry at their parents for having given permission for it.[94] By contrast, the Royal Australasian College of Physicians discloses that "[s]ome men strongly resent having been circumcised as infants."[353] The AAP does not want boys and

350 Frisch M, Simonsen J. Cultural Background, Non-Therapeutic Circumcision and the Risk of Meatal Stenosis and Other Urethral Stricture Disease: Two Nationwide Register-Based Cohort Studies in Denmark 1977–2013. *The Surgeon.* 2018;16:108.

351 Darby RJL. The Sorcerer's Apprentice: Why Can't We Stop Circumcising Boys? *Contexts.* 2005;4:34,37.

352 AAP Speaking Points, falsely claiming, "Isolated cases of morbidity and mortality after ritual circumcision have been reported in the U.S., [but they] have been related to circumcisions that were not performed under sterile conditions."

353 The Royal Australasian College of Physicians. Circumcision of Infant Males. 2010-09. <racp.edu.au/docs/default-source/advocacy-library/circumcision-of-infant-males.pdf>.

men, parents, and the American public to know that circumcision can cause boys and men significant mental distress, both short-term and long-term, or that parents might come to regret having chosen to have their son circumcised.

NOT A HARMLESS SNIP OF A USELESS PIECE OF SKIN

The American Academy of Pediatrics and physicians who circumcise say virtually nothing about the anatomy and physiology of the foreskin, so they portray circumcision as the harmless and painless snip of a useless piece of skin.

The AAP's 2012 policy statement and physicians who circumcise do not disclose that male genital cutting is harmful, even though pain, the loss of the foreskin, and a scar constitute harms.[94]

The AAP claims that circumcision does not appear to adversely affect penile sexual function.[347] That claim is knowingly false, as removing the foreskin plainly destroys its ability to fold and unfold, which stimulates nerves, generates pleasurable sensations, and facilitates comfortable sexual intercourse.

Nor can the AAP prove its claim in 2012 that circumcision "does not appear to adversely affect penile sexual ... sensitivity."[347] It has been known since ancient times that the foreskin is erogenous – Maimonides opined that it should be removed to reduce lust – and physicians knew that it was erogenous in the late 1800s when they introduced it to prevent masturbation. Any male who has a foreskin knows that it is erogenous, and studies, which the AAP does not disclose or rebut, show that it is the most sensitive part of the penis.

The AAP has not provided any evidence or metric to quantify its claim that circumcision does not reduce sexual sensitivity, and that claim contradicts the AAP's statement in 1999 that it might.[348] At a 2013 debate, when asked how removing the highly innervated and mobile foreskin could not affect penile function and sensitivity, Dr. Brady replied, "The question is, then, are the other portions of the penis capable of providing accommodation to maintain the same level of sensitivity and function? ... [T]here's no evidence that there is a valid loss ... there wouldn't be a loss ... it turns out that we can't identify a loss."[235] Thus, Dr. Brady admits that circumcision removes nerves, and essentially admits that this is a loss or harm, but he claims that somehow other parts of the penis make up for the loss, though the AAP does not know how it does so.[235] This is another example of the junk science that the American medical profession has used to try to justify this practice for the past 150 years.

CHAPTER SUMMARY

- The 2012 circumcision policy statement of the American Academy of Pediatrics falsely claims that circumcision is not bad for health.
- The policy statement does not disclose that circumcision is not medically necessary, which parents may not realize.
- The AAP misleadingly describes circumcision as common and simple.
- The AAP knows that operators are often not well trained, and that often anesthetic is not used.
- The AAP cannot prove its claim that pain is well tolerated when anesthetic is used.
- The AAP falsely claims that circumcision is safe when it knows that it is not.
- Overall, the AAP and physicians who perform circumcisions falsely and fraudulently portray circumcision as the common, simple, and safe snip of a useless piece of skin, or nearly so.

21 FRAUDULENT MEDICAL CLAIM: GOOD FOR HEALTH

As discussed in Chapter 9 (Physicians Bear the Burden of Justifying Genital Cutting), physicians bear the burden of every medical procedure – here, male genital cutting – on medical grounds. The principal defense that the American medical profession has been advancing for the past 150 years is that it is good for the health of boys and men in many ways. Americans have not had the knowledge or any reason to doubt the truth of that claim. As discussed in Chapter 14 (The Past as Prelude to the Present), however, the early claims that it cures or prevents more than one hundred different diseases proved to be false. This suggests that we should be very wary of the claim by the American Academy of Pediatrics in 2012 that new evidence shows that it has an array of medical benefits and that it prevents HIV, our disease du jour.

In addition, as recently as 1999, the American Medical Association wrote that circumcision is not medically justified. The American Academy of Pediatrics must know that it is not medically justified today either. It has never recommended circumcision; in 2012 it wrote that the medical benefits are not great enough to recommend it; and in 2016, a member of the AAP's committee on circumcision wrote that boys are not usually circumcised for medical reasons anyway.

That having been said, what are the AAP's arguments today that male genital cutting is good for health, and do their arguments justify the practice? The answer is "no."

FALSE CLAIM THAT CIRCUMCISION HAS AN ARRAY OF "MEDICAL BENEFITS"

In the face of declining circumcision rates and revenues, the American Academy of Pediatrics claimed for the first time in its 2012 guidelines that the practice has actual medical benefits.

> Evaluation of current evidence indicates that the *health benefits* of newborn male circumcision outweigh the risks; furthermore, the benefits of newborn male circumcision justify access to this

> procedure for families who choose it. *Specific benefits* from male circumcision were identified for the prevention of urinary tract infections, acquisition of HIV, transmission of some sexually transmitted infections, and penile cancer (emphasis added).[347]

The AAP also claimed in the 2012 guidelines that the *benefits* outweigh the risks. The widely publicized claim, then, is that circumcision has actual benefits: it will benefit every boy and man.

This claim is knowingly false and intended to deceive the public and parents. Removing the foreskin of the penis does not prevent urinary tract infections, penile cancer, or sexually transmitted infections including HIV. Circumcised males can still contract these diseases. The AAP knows that, as it previously claimed only that circumcision has *potential medical benefits,* meaning slightly reduced risks.[348] The AAP's technical report, submitted to support the guidelines, only talks about reduced risks, or potential medical benefits, not about actual benefits.

This is fraudulent. The 1978 case of *Simcuski v. Saeli* is on point.[354] There, the New York Court of Appeals held that a physician had falsely and fraudulently assured the plaintiff that a treatment had been effective. The AAP and physicians who circumcise can be held liable for falsely and knowingly claiming that circumcision *prevents* a wide array of diseases, when the truth is that it does not prevent any of them.

UNPROVEN CLAIM THAT IT EVEN HAS "POTENTIAL MEDICAL BENEFITS"

The AAP's real claim in 1989, 1999, and 2012 is not that circumcision has actual medical benefits but rather that it has "potential medical benefits." Even if parents are told that circumcision has potential medical benefits during *The Talk*, however, they may not realize that a potential medical benefit is not an actual benefit. Moreover, the claim by a physician that circumcision has potential medical benefits makes it sound as if the potential medical benefits are significant, or a reason to elect circum-

---

354 Simcuski v. Saeli, 377 N.E. 2d 713 (N.Y. 1978). <scholar.google.com/scholar_case?case=16340784914761444812>.

cision, but physicians and the AAP do not give the parents any numbers to go by.

What, then, are these supposedly valuable potential medical benefits? According to the AAP in its widely publicized 2012 circumcision guidelines, which the AAP has not renounced, circumcising 100 boys will prevent one urinary tract infection (UTI); circumcising between 909 and 322,000 newborn boys will prevent one case of penile cancer[347,355] (by comparison, the chance of being hit by lightning is around 1 in 500,000); and circumcising 38 million men in Africa will prevent HIV in 567,166 men there.

The AAP has not proven any of these claims to be true, however. As Matthew Giannetti wrote in 1999, the UTI studies that the AAP invoked were methodologically flawed,[347] and the AAP knew it. There are no randomized controlled trials linking UTIs to circumcision status.[6] The Cochrane Review has determined that "circumcision cannot be shown to meaningfully lessen the risk of contracting a UTI."[356] European medical experts write that "UTI incidence does not seem to be lower in the United States."[6] Thus, the oft touted claim that circumcision reduces the risk of UTIs by 1% is unproven. As to penile cancer, European medical experts write, "It is remarkable that incidence rates of penile cancer in the United States, where ~75% of the non-Jewish, non-Muslim male population is circumcised, are similar to rates in northern Europe, where ≤10% of the male population is circumcised."[6] It is therefore unproven whether circumcision reduces the risk of penile cancer. In addition, there has been no randomized controlled trial, the gold standard of medical evidence, linking neonatal circumcision in the United States with a reduction in HIV in the U.S. And as discussed below, a recent large study in Canada suggests that circumcision does not reduce the risk of HIV at all. Thus, the AAP's central medical claims in 2012 that circumcision might slightly reduce the risk of UTIs, penile cancer, and HIV in the U.S. are *all unproven.*

---

355 Assoc. of Am. Phys. & Surg. v. Weinberger, 395 F. Supp. 125, 129–30 (N.D. Ill. 1975).
356 Svoboda JS. Nontherapeutic Circumcision of Minors as an Ethically Problematic Form of Iatrogenic Injury. *AMA J Ethics.* 2017;19(8):815-824, at n. 30. <journalofethics.ama-assn.org/article/nontherapeutic-circumcision-minors-ethically-problematic-form-iatrogenic-injury/2017-08>.

Little Prospect of Benefiting Any Boy or Man

There is no need to debate these scientific claims, however. Let us assume that the AAP's claims are true. Americans are unlikely to realize the implication, that circumcision has little prospect of benefiting any boy or man. Granting the AAP's claims, it would be necessary to expose one hundred boys to the risks and harms of genital surgery to prevent a single UTI; up to 322,000 newborn boys to prevent a single case of penile cancer;[347] and 67 men to prevent one case of HIV in African men.

Importantly, physicians are not allowed to operate on a person when, as here, it is unlikely to benefit him or her at all. This violates the ethical rule of beneficence, whereby every medical intervention must do good for or benefit each patient.

Boys Are Not at Risk of Adult Diseases

Parents and the American public also may not realize that the only potential medical benefit claimed in childhood is a 1% reduction in UTIs. Most potential medical benefits claimed for the operation accrue in adulthood (e.g., reduction in penile cancer and STIs). But *newborn boys and older boys are not at risk of adult diseases.* As European medical experts write, adult diseases "do not represent compelling reasons for surgery before boys are old enough to decide for themselves."[347] Circumcision thus "fails to meet the commonly accepted criteria for the justification of preventive medical procedures in children."[347] These experts write,

> [F]rom an HIV prevention perspective, if at all effective in a Western context, circumcision can wait until boys are old enough to engage in sexual relationships. Boys can decide for themselves, therefore, whether they want to get circumcised to obtain, at best, partial protection against HIV or rather remain genitally intact and adopt safe-sex practices that are far more effective. ... Not only can circumcision wait, but in order to respect boys' right to self-determination, physicians must wait and defer circumcision until adulthood.[6]

THERE ARE FAR BETTER WAYS TO PREVENT THESE DISEASES

As these European medical experts write, "The cardinal medical question should not be whether circumcision can prevent disease, but how disease can best be prevented." For example, if a person injures a leg, it is better to treat the injury than to amputate the leg. To do otherwise would violate the ethical rule of proportionality, whereby physicians must recommend the optimal treatment for any medical problem, the one that does the most to improve health and the least to harm it. (The rule of proportionality is a legal principle as well. For example, it is part of the international and U.S. laws of war.[357,358])

Urinary tract infections can be treated easily with antibiotics. Penile cancer can be avoided by washing the penis. The AAP knows this as it stated in 1975, "A program of education leading to continuing good personal hygiene would offer all the advantages of circumcision without the attendant surgical risk."[286] Sexually transmitted infections can be avoided by monogamy and using condoms, which are highly effective. The American Medical Association was correct when it wrote in 1999 that it is irresponsible to promote circumcision as a preventative measure against sexually transmitted diseases. Since it is possible to avoid these diseases without the risks and harms of circumcision surgery, there is no valid medical reason to perform the operation. Thus, *circumcision has no medical benefit or advantage.* Circumcision has only disadvantages and no advantages.

As mentioned in the Prologue, penile cancer sounded like a very frightening disease to me. Telling parents that circumcision prevents or reduces the risk of UTIs, penile cancer, and HIV are all scare tactics designed to sell this lucrative unnecessary surgery to unsuspecting parents.

357 Fundamental principles of IHL [International Humanitarian Law], How Does Law Protect in War? <casebook.icrc.org/glossary/fundamental-principles-ihl>.

358 The rule of proportionality is mentioned in the Department of Defense Law of War Manual (June 2015) 304 times. <dod.defense.gov/Portals/1/Documents/pubs/DoD%20Law%20of%20War%20Manual%20-%20June%202015%20Updated%20Dec%202016.pdf?ver=2016-12-13-172036-190>.

FRAUDULENT CLAIM THAT REDUCES THE RISK OF HIV BY 60% IN THE U.S.

A centerpiece of the AAP's 2012 guidelines is the widely publicized claim that circumcision reduces the risk of males contracting HIV during heterosexual sex with HIV infected females by 60%. The claim is based on randomized clinical trials on men in Africa.

Hill and Boyle showed in the Journal of Law and Medicine in 2011,[359] however, that those trials were seriously flawed:

> While the 'gold standard' for medical trials is the randomised, double-blind, placebo-controlled trial, the African trials suffered design and sampling problems ... Several factors may jeopardise the internal validity of [the trials], including: researcher expectation bias; participant expectation bias; inadequate double blinding; lead-time bias; selection and sampling bias; experimental mortality; and early termination.[359]

Thus, the biases that circumcision advocates have in favor of circumcision, discussed in Chapter 15 (Undisclosed Conflicts of Interest and Motives to Defraud), extend into even into randomized controlled trials. The problems with the African studies were so numerous and serious that it was unproven and in serious doubt in 2012 whether circumcision does reduce HIV by 60% even among men in Africa. Let us assume again, though, that the claim is true. Hill and Boyle wrote in 2011,

> What does the frequently cited '60% relative reduction' in HIV infections actually mean? Across all three female-to-male trials, of the 5,411 men subjected to male circumcision, 64 (1.18%) became HIV-positive. Among the 5,497 controls, 137 (2.49%) became HIV-positive, so the absolute decrease in HIV

---

359 Boyle GJ, Hill G. Sub-Saharan African Randomised Clinical Trials into Male Circumcision and HIV Transmission: Methodological, Ethical and Legal Concerns. *J L Med.* 2011-12;19(2):316-34. <pubmed.ncbi.nlm.nih.gov/22320006>.

infection was only 1.31%, which is not statistically signifi-cant.[359]

The claim that circumcision reduces HIV by an impressive sounding 60% must have been intended to mislead the American public and African men because it represents the *relative risk reduction*. (Incidentally, an African man writes, "Do you know why most of us got circumcised here? It's because of the goodies organizations came with, things like sugar, salt, mosquito nets and cooking oil." That is to say, the men were not enthusiastic about being circumcised and had to be bribed.) 60% fewer men became HIV positive. But the *absolute risk reduction* was only 1.3%. If one hundred men were circumcised, then, it would prevent 1.3 men on average from getting HIV, for a short period of time. The AAP's claim "reduces HIV by 60%!" sells circumcision whereas "reduces HIV by 1.3%!" would fall on deaf ears. Even granting the AAP's claim of an absolute 1.3% risk reduction in HIV in Africa,[359] where the prevalence of HIV is high, the absolute risk reduction would be much lower in the U.S.[360] In addition, the number of men who contract HIV from heterosexual sex in the U.S. is low as most men in the U.S. contract HIV from sex with men and from HIV infected needles.

The American Academy of Pediatrics also limited its discussion to studies of African men, while ignoring completed studies performed in North America.[361] None of the studies in North America found that circumcision significantly reduces the risk of HIV infection.[362,363,364] Shortly before the release of the AAP's 2012 guidelines, one study from

360 Personal communication from Robert S. Van Howe, M.D.

361 Laumann, EO, Masi CM, Zuckerman EW. Circumcision in the United States: Prevalence, Prophylactic Effects, and Sexual Practice. *JAMA*. 1997-04-02;277(13):1052-7. Finding "no significant differences between circumcised and uncircumcised men in their likelihood of contracting sexually transmitted diseases." <cirp.org/library/general/laumann>.

362 Mor Z, et al. Declining Rates in Male Circumcision amidst Increasing Evidence of its Public Health Benefit. *PLOS One*. 2007;2:e861. <journals.plos.org/plosone/article?id=10.1371/journal.pone.0000861>.

363 Thomas AG, et al. Prevalence of Circumcision and Its Association With HIV and Sexually Transmitted Infections in A Male US Navy Population. *Naval Health Res Ctr*. 2004-07;04(10).

364 Warner L, et al. Male Circumcision and Risk of HIV Infection among Heterosexual African American Men Attending Baltimore Sexually Transmitted Disease Clinics. *J Infect Dis*. 2009-01-01;199:59.

Puerto Rico, which the AAP did not disclose, found that circumcised men were at significantly greater risk of HIV than intact men.[365]

Even if the unproven claim were true that circumcision reduces the risk of HIV by 1.3% (actually, less) in the United States, heterosexually active males are at risk of contracting it whether they are circumcised or not. They would therefore still need to be monogamous, avoid unsafe sexual partners, or use a condom. Hill and Boyle wrote, "'Condom use after male circumcision is essential for HIV prevention.' What is the purpose of male circumcision, if condom use is still needed to prevent sexual transmission of HIV?"[359] Thus, even granting all claims, circumcision has no value in reducing the risk of HIV.

The AAP should be warning all men *against* getting circumcised because it does not prevent HIV; because it is unproven whether it even slightly reduces the risk (in Africa, let alone in the U.S.); and because much more effective, non-invasive, painless, risk free, and less expensive alternatives are readily available, without the loss of the foreskin. These include limiting exposure to infected sexual partners, pre-exposure prophylaxis, and condoms.[366] The AAP's report does not even mention condoms. Mentioning HIV is another scare tactic like mentioning penile cancer, and an effective one.

In September 2021, The Journal of Urology published the most extensive study of HIV and circumcision ever completed, "Circumcision and risk of HIV among males from Ontario, Canada."[367] The study examined 570,000 males born in Ontario who underwent circumcision at any age between 1991 and 2017. The results suggest that circumcision provides no protective effect in North America against contracting HIV. Although the study does not provide conclusive proof of that, it is evidence that circumcision is not associated with lower HIV rates. If the AAP were honest, it would disclose this study to the public, as it brings into serious

---

365 Rodriguez-Diaz CE, et al. More than Foreskin: Circumcision Status, History of HIV/STI, and Sexual Risk in a Clinic-Based Sample of Men in Puerto Rico. *J Sex Med.* 2012-08;9(11):2933. <researchgate.net/publication/230684293>.

366 HIV Basics, Prevention, U.S. Centers For Disease Control and Prevention. <cdc.gov/hiv/basics/prevention.html>.

367 Nayan M, Hamilton RJ, Juurlink DN, Austin PC, Jarvi KA. Circumcision and risk of HIV among males from Ontario, Canada. *J Urology.* 2021-09. <arclaw.org/wp-content/uploads/Nayan-Circumcision-and-Risk-of-HIV-Among-Males-from-Ontario-Canada-J-Urology-2021.pdf>.

doubt the validity of the AAP's widely publicized and central claim in 2012 that circumcision reduces the risk of HIV.

The AAP also forgot to inform the public that "[i]n the Ugandan male-to-female trial, there appears to have been a 61% relative *increase* in HIV infection among female partners of HIV-positive circumcised men (emphasis added)." The AAP should be warning women about this increase instead of hiding the fact. And since any reduction in HIV in men is offset by an equal increase in women, there is no net gain in reducing HIV by circumcising the men.

FRAUDULENT CLAIM THAT "THE BENEFITS OUTWEIGH THE RISKS"

The public and the parents of newborn boys will have no reason to doubt the truth of this claim either,[94] another centerpiece of the AAP's now-expired 2012 circumcision statement, but it is indefensible. 1) When circumcision seriously injures or kills a boy, the benefits do not outweigh the risks. 2) The AAP never made this claim before 2012; it is the only national-level pediatric society in the world to have made this claim; and it employed no recognized method of weighing or balancing either benefits or risks.[368] 3) The AAP stated in its 2012 technical report that "The true incidence of complications after newborn circumcision is unknown."[94] Since the AAP admits that it does not know the incidence of risks, it cannot logically conclude or believe its claim that the benefits outweigh the risks. Moreover, in 2013, the AAP backpedaled, writing, "These benefits were *felt* to outweigh the risks of the procedure" (emphasis added).[94] That is speculation, not science. 4) A 2021 study shows that circumcision causes meatal stenosis, a narrowing of the urethral opening, in 17.9% of cases.[369] Thus, circumcision causes infections about eighteen more times than it prevents a urinary tract infection, and UTIs can be treated with antibiotics. 5) Importantly, the AAP assigned no value to the foreskin and thus left it out of the equation, despite its manifestly special importance to males.[103]

368 AAP Task Force on Circumcision 2012. The AAP Task Force on Neonatal Circumcision: a call for respectful dialogue. *J Med Ethics.* 2013;39:1. <jme.bmj.com/content/39/7/442>.
369 Acimi S, et al. Prevalence and causes of meatal stenosis in circumcised boys. *J Pediatr Urol.* 2022-02;18(1):89.e1-6. <pubmed.ncbi.nlm.nih.gov/34740536>.

The truth is that it is circumcision is harmful and risky on the one hand with little prospect of any medical benefit on the other hand, and any benefits can be achieved without it. Thus, circumcision has only disadvantages and no advantages.

A European physician writes: "[T]he [AAP's] claim, that there are health benefits in excising a piece of healthy tissue from the penis of a healthy neonate, is as absurd as would be the claim that amputating the left little finger of a neonate has health benefits. In this European physician's view, the U.S. practice of circumcising healthy newborn (and older) boys is crazy."[370]

CHAPTER SUMMARY

- American medical associations, physicians, and hospitals defraud the public by implying and by expressly claiming that circumcision is good for health.
- They falsely claim that it has actual medical benefits, when it has little prospect of benefiting any boy or man.
- The American Academy of Pediatrics has not met its burden of proving its longstanding claims that male genital cutting reduces the risk of UTIs, penile cancer, and STIs including HIV.
- A 2021 study suggests that circumcision has no protective effect against HIV.
- The AAP has hidden the fact that circumcision may increase the acquisition of HIV by females by the same amount that it decreases HIV in men, so there is no net gain in the reduction of HIV.
- Boys are not at risk of adult diseases, so they are not a valid medical reason to circumcise boys. If men want to be circumcised, they can choose it for themselves.
- Even if circumcision has any potential medical benefits, which is unproven, they all can be achieved safely and much more easily and effectively without the risks and harms of the operation. Thus, circumcision has no medical benefits. There is no medical reason to choose it.

370 Lindahl HG. European Doctors Say, "Routine Circumcision is Insane." *Intaction.* 2013-01-22. <intaction.org/european-doctors-say-routine-circumcision-is-insane>.

- The American medical profession assigns no value to the foreskin, even though adolescent boys and men who have one do.
- The AAP's claim that "the benefits outweigh the risks" is false and fraudulent.

22   Fraudulent Legal Claims

As background, the American Academy of Pediatrics made unsustainable legal claims in the past in the context of female genital cutting.[371] It once appeared to condone physicians performing a ritual clitoral nick of a girls' genitals if a girl's parents requested it. This would have violated girls' rights, including state statutes prohibiting female genital cutting except when medically necessary.[371] Facing a firestorm of criticism, the AAP quickly retired the guideline.[372] Thus, the AAP promoted female genital cutting – though the least harmful form of it – even in the face of a federal law forbidding it. As discussed below, the AAP's legal advice about male genital cutting cannot be trusted either.[372]

"Physicians Have the Right to Operate On a Healthy Child"

It is self-evident that physicians are only licensed and allowed to practice medicine. Thus, it is a knowingly false legal claim for the American medical profession to claim, expressly and by implication, that physicians have the right to operate on a perfectly healthy child, and thus without a valid diagnosis and without a recommendation that the child needs an operation. The AAP must be aware of the legal scholarship showing that circumcision is unlawful and indeed criminal child abuse, and it is aware of the German court ruling that it is a crime for a physician to circumcise a boy for religious reasons. The AAP has not come close to refuting the claim that circumcision is unlawful and child abuse.

Physicians might argue that they are not familiar with the law, and that they do not know that circumcision is unlawful. That argument fails, however, because the legal and ethical rules about circumcision are the same. Physicians are required to be familiar with the rules of medical ethics. They certainly know that they are not allowed to harm a patient,

371 American Academy of Pediatrics. Policy Statement – Ritual Genital Cutting of Female Minors. *Pediatrics.* 2010-05;125(5):1088-93, p. 1092.
<publications.aap.org/pediatrics/article/125/5/1088/72431/Ritual-Genital-Cutting-of-Female-Minors>.

372 Louden K. AAP Retracts Controversial Policy on Female Genital Cutting. *Medscape Med News.* 2010-06-02. <medscape.com/viewarticle/722840>.

that they must respect each patient's autonomy, and that they are not allowed to enrich themselves at the expense of their patient.

"PARENTS HAVE THE RIGHT TO ELECT IT"

Since 1975, shortly after the stating in 1971 that there is no medical indication for circumcision during the newborn period,[373] the AAP has claimed that parents have the unrestricted right to elect it. The AAP has never cited any legal authority for the claim, however, which it must do to prove that there is such a right. The unsubstantiated claim is a non-starter.

At a 2013 debate about the ethics and legality of the practice, for example, Michael Brady of the AAP's 2012 committee merely argued that there is no law on the books in the U.S. expressly prohibiting circumcision, and that no physician has ever been held liable for a properly performed circumcision.[235] There was no law on the books in Germany prohibiting circumcision before 2012, however, when a court ruled that it constitutes criminal assault: the crime simply had not previously been prosecuted.

At the debate, Attorney J. Steven Svoboda made a compelling case that circumcision violates numerous rights of the child. Against this, I recall that the committee's ethicist, Douglas Diekema, said the next day that the American Academy of Pediatrics rejects the children's rights-based view of circumcision,[235] without giving any reason in support of that claim. Thus, in the AAP's view, children do not have any of the rights enumerated and cited in Chapter 6 (Adults' and Children's Rights). Dr. Diekema, a physician, ethicist, and scholar, knows that autonomy is a fundamental rule of medical ethics,[187] and his claim is indefensible. The right of every person to an intact body and to decide its fate is an "inalienable" or absolute and fundamental under U.S. law and in common law countries.[374] Dr. Diekema himself wrote early that older children and adolescents should not be circumcised in the face of dissent,[212] implicitly

---

373 1971 AAP Statement. <cirp.org/library/statements/aap/#a1971>.
374 Equal and Inalienable Rights. *Documents of Freedom.*
   <web.archive.org/web/20210418115739/https://www.docsoffreedom.org/student/readings/
   equal-and-inalienable-rights>.

recognizing that older children have some rights when it comes to circumcision, namely the right to object. The U.S. Centers for Disease Control & Prevention also correctly observed in 2018, "Delaying male circumcision until adolescence or adulthood obviates concerns about violation of autonomy."[375] Thus, the CDC also knows that non-therapeutic circumcision violates the child's right to autonomy.

As the U.S. Congress stated regarding female genital cutting,[376] and as the German court held in 2012, boys' right to intact genitalia supersedes their parents' religious and other rights.[231] The United States Supreme Court has recognized this as well. In 1979 in *Parham v. J.R.,* the Court ruled that although parents have responsibility for the upbringing of their child, a child has a liberty interest in not being confined unnecessarily for medical treatment, in that case for mental illness. Although parents may seek to institutionalize a child for mental illness, children should only be institutionalized when there is an independent medical determination that the child needs to be.[377]

Thus, the AAP has never responded in any meaningful way to the arguments by legal scholars dating back to 1985 that male genital cutting is child abuse and unlawful,[203] nor to the German ruling that circumcision is a crime.[231] The AAP has ignored the legal controversy. Similarly, despite nearly 100 publications available in 2012 addressing the substantial ethical issues associated with non-therapeutic circumcision, the AAP's 2012 Task Force did not seriously address the ethical controversy either. It likely did not do so because there is no defense to the accusation that forced genital cutting is unethical and unlawful. It can be inferred that the American medical profession does not want the public to know that there is even any question about whether circumcision is ethical and legal.

---

375 Background, Methods, and Synthesis of Scientific Information Used to Inform "Information for Providers to Share with Male Patients and Parents Regarding Male Circumcision and the Prevention of HIV Infection, Sexually Transmitted Infections, and other Health Outcomes". 2018-08-22;1-82, p. 49. <stacks.cdc.gov/view/cdc/58457>.
376 Belluck P. Federal Ban on Female Genital Mutilation Ruled Unconstitutional by Judge. *NY Times.* 2018-11-21. <nytimes.com/2018/11/21/health/fgm-female-genital-mutilation-law.html>.
377 Parham v. J.R., 442 U.S. 584, 585 (1979). <scholar.google.com/scholar_case?case=15981297995569250470>.

"Parents Will Need to Weigh Their Own Religious, Cultural, and Personal Aesthetic Preferences In Doing So"

The AAP has also long claimed, without citing a single statute or case in support of the proposition, that it is legitimate for parents to take various non-medical factors into consideration in making the circumcision decision.[94] These include the climate;[286] parents' religious, cultural, and personal aesthetic preferences (looking like daddy);[378] "the social and emotional reaction of prospective parents to penile cleansing, and the ability to understand and facilitate good hygiene" if circumcision is not elected;[378] and even social pressures.[85] The AAP's 2012 guidelines state:

> Parents ultimately should decide whether circumcision is in the best interests of their male child. They *will need to* weigh medical information in the context of their own religious, ethical, and cultural beliefs and practices. The medical benefits alone may not outweigh these other considerations for individual families (emphasis added).[94]

It is absurd for physicians to take any of these factors into account as none of them have anything to do with the child's health or with medicine. In its 2019 circumcision guidelines, the British Medical Association advises its physicians to, "be alert to situations in which parents' decisions appear to be contrary to their child's interests."[178]

Since physicians do not ask parents why they choose to have their son circumcised, the American Academy of Pediatrics is also falsely implying that parents have the unfettered right to elect to have their son's genitals cut for any reason or for no reason.[297] Physicians and the AAP therefore condone even so-called "spite circumcisions," where a malevolent father wants to circumcise the son to spite the mother.[379] They also condone circumcising boys who say they do not want to be circumcised. In sharp

---

378 Freedman AL. Circumcision Debate: Beyond Benefits and Risks. See note #71.

379 See, e.g., the Hironimus case in Florida: Freeman M. Mom Signs Consent for Son's Circumcision to Get Out of Jail – but Now Faces New Criminal Charge. *Sun Sentinel.* 2015-05-22.<sun-sentinel.com/local/palm-beach/fl-circumcision-mother-court-hearing-20150522-story.html>.

contrast, the British Medical Association states that "the BMA cannot envisage a situation in which it is ethically acceptable to circumcise a child or young person who refuses the procedure, irrespective of the parents' wishes."[178]

Just as most parents know little or nothing about medicine and have no reason or ability to question the AAP's medical claims, they know little or nothing about the law and they have no reason or ability to question the AAP's legal claims. By contrast, the AAP's 2012 committee included a lawyer, and the AAP has access to the country's finest lawyers.[380] As discussed in Chapter 6 (Adults' and Children's Rights), parents do not own their children, however, and the claim that parents can do whatever they want to their children's bodies as if they own their child's body is a dead dogma.[204]

The federal government, state governments, and courts recognize that parents "may at times be acting against the interests of their children."[381] Otherwise there would be no need for the child abuse statutes. American Medical Association Opinion 2.2.1 gives parents further guidance: "[i]n giving or withholding permission for medical *treatment* for their children, parents/guardians are expected to safeguard their children's physical health and well-being and to nurture their children's developing personhood and autonomy."[166] Thus, parents, like physicians, have a legal duty to respect their child's autonomy and do what is best for their child's health, without regard to their own personal preferences if different.

Accordingly, the AAP's long standing claim that parents have the unfettered right to elect to have their healthy son circumcised is knowingly false and fraudulent.[94] Parents are only allowed to give permission for an operation on their child when their child needs the operation and it cannot be deferred.[292] In fact, in Germany, parents who give permission to have their healthy son circumcised unwittingly commit the crime of assault themselves.[231] In the U.S. as well, not only performing but also authorizing a circumcision constitute criminal child abuse and a civil battery.

---

380 2012 AAP Technical Report, p. e778 (noting that the task force included Steven Wegner, MD, JD). *Pediatrics.* 2012. <pediatrics.aappublications.org/content/pediatrics/130/3/e756.pdf>.
381 Bartley v. Kremens, 402 F. Supp. 1039, 1047-48 (1975), vacated and remanded, 431 U. S. 119 (1977).

"Circumcision Is a Religious Right"

The American Academy of Pediatrics and physicians who circumcise also claim that parents have the right to elect circumcision for religious reasons. If the AAP were neutral, it would inform parents that Christian and Catholic doctrine oppose circumcision. In a lawsuit, *Marriage of Boldt,* several Jewish organizations similarly claimed that parents have a religious right to elect circumcision under the First Amendment Freedom of Religion clause.[382] They wanted a Jewish father to be able to have his son circumcised, even over the objection of the mother and the boy. It is certainly important to determine whether parents do have this right, as claimed, to have their son circumcised for religious reasons.

It is granted that in America, considerable deference is given to religion. Nonetheless, there is no such religious right to intrude into another person's body, as the European cases and the U.S. law cited above conclusively show.[231] This result does not stem from any animus toward religious adherents, many of whom sincerely believe that it is a religious requirement and tradition to circumcise boys.[383] Rather, it stems from the fact that constitutional rights are personal. Only individuals have constitutional rights, and they exist only for the benefit of the individual. A person's constitutional rights do not extend to allowing him or her to inflict bodily harm on another person's body.[141] Merkel and Putzke write, "No conceivable (positive) liberty right, roughly understood as a right to perform certain acts at one's will, can possibly justify direct physical intrusion into someone else's body."[141] There is no legal support for the often repeated claim by the American medical profession and by religious adherents that parents have the religious right to elect to have their son circumcised.

---

382 Boldt v. Boldt, 176 P.3d 388 (Or. 2008), cert. denied, 555 U.S. 814 (2008). <scholar.google.com/scholar_case?case=15733935640861799 97>. Thus, Jewish organizations want Jewish fathers to be able to elect to have their son circumcised even when the son and mother do not want it. We note parenthetically that boys circumcised for religious reasons are exposed to the same risks and suffer the harms as all circumcised boys and the men they become.

383 Scholz KA. Circumcision Remains Legal in Germany. *DW.* 2012-12-12. <dw.com/en/circumcision-remains-legal-in-germany/a-16399336>.

To the contrary, children and the adults they become have their own right or freedom to choose their parents' religion, a different religion, or no religion.[141] Since parents do not have a right to determine their son's religious affiliation for his lifetime, they do not have a right to permanently mark their children's bodies with a symbol of that affiliation either.[141] In the U.S. as in Germany,[231] such a mark violates the boys' rights to bodily integrity, self-determination and privacy, and freedom of religion, which supersede their parents' religious and other rights.[384]

For example, when the U.S. Congress banned female genital cutting (ignoring that a federal court subsequently ruled that federal statute unconstitutional), it also found correctly that such a ban does not violate any person's rights under the First Amendment, referring to the Freedom of Religion clause. The same is true of male genital cutting, which as shown is analogous to female genital cutting.

Directly on point, the U.S. Supreme Court ruled in *Prince v. Massachusetts* in 1944 that parents are not allowed to expose their children to the risk of physical or psychological harm, let alone to actually harm them (as male genital cutting does), based on the parents' religious beliefs.[385] The court in *Prince* famously stated that parents may martyr themselves, but not their children.[385] Merkel and Putzke write that insofar as circumcision is more than merely a religious rite, but a significant bodily harm to the child, it is inevitable that this "brings the law onto the scene."[141]

The American Academy of Pediatrics knows that its legal claim that parents have the religious right to elect circumcision is false. In 1997, the AAP's own Committee on Bioethics published an article, "Religious Objections to Medical Care" in the AAP's in-house journal *Pediatrics* that concluded:

> The American Academy of Pediatrics (AAP) believes that all
> children deserve effective medical treatment that is likely to

---

384 18 U.S.C. § 116(c) (2012). See note #259. The federal U.S. female genital mutilation statute similarly states that it is of no account if any person believes that the operation is required as a matter of custom or ritual.

385 Prince v. Massachusetts, 21 U.S. 158, 169-70 (1944). <scholar.google.com/scholar_case?case=30125822275354260465>.

prevent substantial harm or suffering or death ... Constitutional guarantees of freedom of religion do not permit children to be harmed through religious practices, nor do they allow religion to be a valid legal defense when an individual harms or neglects a child.[386]

The AAP's Committee on Bioethics even cited the *Prince* case referenced above, as well as the United Nations Convention on the Rights of the Child, in support of its conclusion.[386] The AAP also called for those entrusted with the care of children to "support the repeal of religious exemption laws,"[386] thus including the state statutes that exempt circumcision from prosecution as a form of ritual abuse.

"PHYSICIANS ARE ALLOWED TO TAKE ORDERS FROM PARENTS TO CIRCUMCISE BOYS FOR NON-MEDICAL REASONS"

According to the American Academy of Pediatrics in 2012, in deciding whether or not to elect circumcision, parents will need to take into consideration their own religious, cultural, and personal aesthetic preferences. The claim is, then, that physicians are allowed to take orders from parents to cut off part of their son's penis for reasons having nothing to do with medicine. There is no legal support for this claim either: it is another non-starter.

Even if parents had the right to elect circumcision for non-medical reasons, which they do not, physicians are only licensed to practice medicine. Their job is to serve each pediatric patients' medical needs and to safeguard each patient's health.[386] The AAP knows that physicians are not allowed to take orders from parents to cut boys' genitals for reasons having nothing to do with medicine. Once again, the AAP's own Committee on Bioethics made this clear, in 1995:

Thus 'proxy consent' poses serious problems for pediatric health care providers. Such providers have legal and ethical

---

386 American Academy of Pediatrics Committee on Bioethics. Religious Objections to Medical Care. *Pediatrics.*1997-02;99(2):279-81. <cirp.org/library/ethics/AAP3>.

duties to their child patients to render competent medical care based on what the patient needs, not what someone else expresses. Although impasses regarding the interests of minors and the expressed wishes of their parents or guardians are rare, *the pediatrician's responsibilities to his or her patient exist independent of parental desires or proxy consent* (emphasis added).[386]

The implied claim that physicians are allowed to take orders from parents to operate on a health child is thus another big lie.

CHAPTER SUMMARY

- The American Academy of Pediatrics once condoned a ritual clitoral nick, which physicians would have been paid to perform, even though that would have violated the federal anti-female genital mutilation statute and similar state statutes.
- The AAP has not responded in any meaningful way to the accusations dating back to 1985 that male genital cutting is unethical and unlawful, that the AAP's 1989 and 1999 guidelines were negligent and possibly intentionally fraudulent, or that its 2012 guidelines contain even more indefensible claims.
- The AAP makes the knowingly false legal claims that parents have the right to elect male circumcision for religious, cultural, and personal reasons, and that physicians are allowed to take orders from parents to perform unnecessary genital surgery on boys for such reasons, which have nothing to do with medicine.

23 FRAUDULENT CONSENT FORMS

As discussed in the foregoing chapter, it is a fraud for physicians to ask parents whether they want to have their son circumcised or not: physicians do not have the right to perform the operation; and parents do not have the right to give permission for it. Nonetheless, because physicians do solicit parental permission and let the parents decide, they have a duty to disclose everything to the parents that might affect the parents' decision. If they do not, the parent(s) and their son have additional claims against the physician for lack of fully informed consent, and hence for an unlawful battery and intentional fraud.

Parents need to be informed, as discussed in this book, that the foreskin is a natural body part, an essential component of perfect health, and very good for health. There is no medical indication or need to remove it; physicians in most countries leave it alone; and no national medical association in the world recommends it. The form would disclose all of the attendant risks and harms, including that the procedure can be fatal and can cause psychological harm, and that it removes the most sensitive part of the penis. Hence, it seriously harms all boys and men. The form would disclose that there is a consensus among courts in Europe and legal scholars that circumcision is unethical and unlawful.

Of course, consent forms do not contain any of this information. As one example, in a Canadian lawsuit, before a mother gave birth, the hospital offered to circumcise the son and "said I needed to have payment ready." The mother testified, "There wasn't a lot of talk about the circumcision more just if I wanted it."[387] As Dr. Diekema stated, half the time parents are not told anything about the operation. The consent form stated that the health care provider informed the mother about the nature of the procedure, the likely outcome, the risks, alternative treatment options, and the consequences of not having the procedure performed. The mother testified on affidavit, however, that the hospital did not discuss any of those things with her. Moreover, whatever it told her orally also should have been written on the consent form. Before her son was born, she asked excellent questions:

---

387 The supporting court documents are available from the author.

> Is circumcision medically necessary and if not, why do you
> offer it? Is it medically justified? Does it hurt? Are there any
> known long-term harms and if so, what are they? Is it in my
> son's best interest? Can there be a psychological impact on my
> son? If it isn't necessary and there aren't good medical reasons
> for it, then why should I give consent instead of my son? And
> are there any parents who regret circumcising their son?[387]

The mother testified in a lawsuit that the nurses were busy and that they only answered a few of her questions. "Before the surgery there was no question period rather the doctor came in, made me sign a form, took the cash and left. The nurses from there took [my son] away to get the procedure done." The hospital responded to her questions twelve days after she gave birth, too late for her to use them, and the answers were all pro-circumcision and evasive. The hospital wrote, "It is not medically necessary however we offer it as an option for parents to get done," without explaining why the hospital offers an unnecessary procedure as an option. The hospital claimed that circumcision "allows for less bacteria and is often the cleaner option in the long run to prevent infections," without disclosing that it is easy to wash the foreskin. "They [falsely] told me there are no long term harms to [my son] as long as the procedure goes according to plan everything will be fine." The hospital thus knew that the procedure could go wrong but did not disclose the nature or frequency of the possible complications to the mother, or that the loss of the foreskin is a long-term harm. "In [the nurse's] experience she has never been told by a parent that they regretted doing a circumcision instead she has had the opposite and most thank her for doing it." Essentially, the hospital told her that there was no risk that she would regret it, but she does. "[The nurses] also said [my son] is too young to remember and that's why they do [circumcisions] at this age so there is no psychological impact on him and that way he won't remember compared to people who get it done later in life." But circumcision at birth can have psychological sequelae, and "won't remember it" is hardly a justification for operating on a child. Another mother informed me, "My sister-in-law years ago was pressured to sign a circumcision consent form at a Catholic hospital in

Buffalo, NY, when a nurse lied and told her she 'had to' sign the consent form. She protected her second son from circumcision."[388]

Consent forms may contain false claims as well. For example, the form for Harvard University's prestigious Brigham and Women's Hospital falsely claims, "there is still some medical controversy about the need for the procedure on a routine basis."[389] The hospital knows that there is no medical need to circumcise boys on a routine basis or at all. The form also falsely states that "the benefits to be reasonably expected compared with alternative approaches have been explained to me," because there are no benefits reasonably to be expected.

The chance of hospitals fully informing parents about circumcision orally or in consent forms must be close to zero. If they did so, most parents would decline the invitation to have their son circumcised. As is happening in Israel, even religious adherents might begin to question the practice. Consent forms will not tell parents the truth about circumcision until legislation forces them to do so.

Chapter Summary

- To be legally valid, circumcision consent forms must disclose everything that might influence a parent's decision, as enumerated above.
- Consent forms do not come close to meeting that legal requirement, so they are legally invalid, and the operation is a battery.
- If consent forms told parents the truth about circumcision, few parents would elect it.
- Fraudulent consent forms are one of the many ways that physicians deceive parents about circumcision and persuade them to elect it.
- Physicians have not told parents the truth about circumcision for the past 150 years, and unless legislation forces them to do so, they never will.

---

388 Personal communication. 2021-08-18.

389 <brighamandwomens.org/assets/BWH/pediatric-newborn-medicine/pdfs/circumcision-consent-form.pdf>.

Of course, money fuels the circumcision industry. When the United Kingdom's National Health Service stopped funding neonatal circumcision in 1950, parents were not willing to pay for it, and the industry there essentially collapsed. In the United States, private insurers reimburse physicians for about two-thirds of all circumcision, while the Medicaid program for the indigent pays for the rest. Thus, if private insurers and/or Medicaid in the U.S. stopped paying for circumcision, the industry would collapse here as well.

As discussed above, physicians are ethically proscribed from performing unnecessary surgery and from billing for it. This is confirmed by a 1956 New York Appellate Division case in which a physician sued a baseball team for the unpaid costs of an operation that he had performed on a baseball player's hand. He claimed that the operation had been unnecessary, and that the physician had intentionally performed it to obtain an unjustified professional fee. The court observed that physicians are not allowed to charge for services that are unnecessary. "[One] need not pay for services that are the result of quackery."[390] The court therefore concluded that physicians who perform unnecessary surgery (and of course charge for it) are quacks. Performing and billing for unnecessary circumcision surgery is indeed quack medicine.

When Blue Cross Blue Shield of Utah was asked in 1994 why it pays for non-therapeutic circumcision, it replied, "It has been known for decades that circumcision provides no demonstrably medically necessary purpose. It is rooted in our culture, however." We pay for it because "the public demands that this service be included in their insurance policy." By contrast, when a member of my family recently was about to undergo surgery, the insurance company explained why it would pay for the surgery: "The decision is based on meeting medical necessity ..." Thus, private insurance companies know that circumcision is not medically necessary, and that they should not be covering it, but they cover it anyway to keep parents (and physicians and hospitals) happy.

---

390 Shenkman v. O'Malley, 2 A.D. 2d 567 (NY App. Div. 1956). <scholar.google.com/scholar_case?case=8385748705989025251>.

The following subpart reprises and builds upon the argument made in a 2011 law review article that it is unlawful for physicians and hospitals in the United States to charge the federal and state Medicaid program for circumcision.[1] It is also unlawful for states to let them get away with it, as thirty-five states and the District of Columbia do.

A CLEAR VIOLATION OF FEDERAL LAW

Under the federal Medicaid Act, 42 U.S.C. § 1396 et seq.,[391] practitioners must furnish only medically necessary care.[392] Physicians must certify that each medical service that they provide is medically indicated or needed, and medically necessary, or the last resort, in order to be reimbursed for it.[393] Numerous U.S. Supreme Court cases state that the purpose of the joint federal and state Medicaid program is to provide federal financial assistance to states that choose to reimburse certain costs of *medically necessary treatment*.[394] Medicaid's purpose is to enable each state to meet the costs of necessary medical services for individuals whose income and resources are insufficient.[395] "Congress has opted to subsidize *medically necessary services* generally" (emphasis added).[396] Federal regulations also require physicians to show evidence of medical necessity for all services provided.[397] Further, every state must establish a utilization review board to review payments in order to reduce unnecessary Medicaid expenditures.[398]

---

391 Harris v. McRae, 448 U.S. 297, 301 (S. Ct. 1980). <scholar.google.com/scholar_case?case=8833310949486291357>.

392 42 C.F.R. § 456.1 (requiring "methods and procedures to safeguard against unnecessary utilization of care and services").

393 42 U.S. Code § 1320c-5 (requiring healthcare providers compensated by Medicaid to show that the procedure is "supported by evidence of medical necessity"); Assoc. of Am. Phys. & Surg. v. Weinberger, 395 F. Supp. 125, 129-30 (N.D. Ill. 1975).

394 Harris v. McRae, 448 U.S. 297, n.1 (1980). The Court used the phrase "medically necessary" 75 times.

395 Schweiker v. Hogan, 457 U.S. 569, 573 (1982), citing 42 U.S.C. § 1396a(a)(10)(C); Beal v. Doe, 432 U.S. 438, 444. (1977). <scholar.google.com/scholar_case?case=4067161982742187409>.

396 Harris v. McRae, 448 U.S. 297, 316-17 (S. Ct. 1980).

397 42 U.S.C. § 1320c-5(a).

398 Emp. of Dep't Pub. Health & Welfare Mo. v. Dep't Pub. Health & Welfare, Mo., 411 U.S. 279 298 (1973). <scholar.google.com/scholar_case?case=16161960573095579546>.

Importantly, by 2011, 18 U.S. states had stopped allowing physicians and hospitals to use Medicaid to pay for non-therapeutic circumcision, whether by legislation or by its Medicaid office giving notice by letter that it is not a covered benefit.[1] Since then, three of the states revived Medicaid coverage so today 15 states and the District of Columbia do not cover it.[399] For example, in 2005 Louisiana "terminated reimbursement for the performance of routine circumcisions of newborn infants and other circumcisions for which medical necessity is not documented." The remaining thirty-five states do not ask physicians and hospitals for evidence of medical necessity or review payments, as required by federal law. If they did, they would determine that most circumcisions are not medically necessary.

A Clear Violation of Every State's Law As Well

Under federal law, every state must require proof of medical necessity and establish a review board to safeguard against paying for unnecessary services. For example, Massachusetts Medicaid regulations only allow payment for inpatient hospital services that are medically necessary.[400] They do not pay a provider for services that are not medically necessary; that are "not reasonably calculated to prevent, diagnose, prevent the worsening of, alleviate, correct, or cure conditions in the member"; or when another comparable but more conservative or less costly alternative exists.[400] In addition, the care must be substantiated by records of medical necessity and must meet professionally recognized standards of health care.[400] Massachusetts law also expressly prohibits using Medicaid to pay for cosmetic surgery, which circumcision is.

Unnecessary genital surgery does not meet any of these requirements for reimbursement in Massachusetts. It is unnecessary; it is performed on

---

399 Arizona since June 5, 2002; California since September 1, 1982; Florida since June 24, 2003; Idaho since March 12, 2005; Louisiana since April 20, 2005; Maine since February 3, 2004; Minnesota since September 1, 2005; Mississippi since August 1, 2000; Montana since January 1, 2003; Nevada since 1999; North Dakota since 1991; Oregon since 1994; South Carolina since February 1, 2011; Utah since March 6, 2003; and Washington since 1999. Research courtesy of Petrina Fadel (Aug. 17, 2021).

400 130 Mass. Code Regs. 450.204 (2020).

boys who are not suffering from any medical condition; it is cosmetic surgery; better alternatives exist; physicians do not substantiate their claims by records of medical necessity; and non-therapeutic circumcision does not meet professionally recognized standards of health care.

Even though male genital cutting manifestly does not qualify for re-imbursement by Medicaid under federal and state laws, physicians and hospitals in 35 U.S. states bill Medicaid for it anyway. They have likely been doing so with impunity dating back to the beginning of the federal program in 1965 or when the state adopted the program, if later. Thus, physicians are committing Medicaid fraud every time they bill the Medic-aid program for circumcising a healthy boy. The U.S. federal government and state governments have claims against physicians who perform cir-cumcisions for potentially billions of dollars for unlawful Medicaid bill-ing,[401] likely dating back to 1965.[401] Instead of forcing physicians and hospitals to comply with the law, however, the federal Medicaid office and the 35 state Medicaid offices turn a blind eye to it and reimburse them anyway.

THE AAP'S SCHEME TO DEFRAUD MEDICAID

The U.S. Government Accountability Office has designated Medicaid as a program that is at "high risk for improper payments," including for those that were not medically necessary.[402] The federal Fifth Circuit has stated where "the government has conditioned payment of a claim upon a claimant's certification of compliance with, for example, a statute or regulation, a claimant submits a false or fraudulent claim when he or she falsely certifies compliance with that statute or regulation."[403]

In *United States v. Laughlin,* the Tenth Circuit held that a person who makes a knowingly false Medicaid claim can be convicted of Medicaid fraud.[404] The American Academy of Ophthalmology acknowledged this

---

401 Id. at 343.
402 Laws Against Health Care Fraud Resource Guide 1 (2014).
403 U.S. ex rel. Marcy v. Rowan, 520 F.3d 384, 389 (5th Cir. 2008; internal quotations omitted): <scholar.google.com/scholar_case?case=6371312137102085736>.
404 United States v. Laughlin, 26 F.3d 1523, 1526 (10th Cir. 1994). <scholar.google.com/scholar_case?case=18298571079617644122>.

when it stated in 2016 that "[c]laiming reimbursement for unnecessary surgery could also constitute fraud under Medicare/Medicaid or private insurance policies."[405]

In addition, it is a violation of 18 U.S.C. § 1347 to knowingly and willfully execute a scheme to defraud any health care benefit program.[406] In *United States v. Bajoghli,* the court held that the owner of a surgery center had engaged in a lucrative fraudulent scheme of performing and billing for unnecessary surgeries.[407]

The American Academy of Pediatrics calls circumcision elective,[94] meaning that it is a choice, and non-therapeutic, meaning not required for therapeutic purposes. Therefore, the AAP knows that these circumcisions are unnecessary. The AAP also observed in 2012 that "more families may be choosing not to have a circumcision because of a sense [actually, a justified true belief, or with knowledge] that it is not medically necessary."[408] In the face of declining Medicaid coverage, declining circumcision rates, and declining revenues, however, the 2012 circumcision policy statement of the AAP nonetheless contains an unprecedented plea for the revival of Medicaid coverage in states that had properly ended it, without giving a reason why physicians should be compensated for performing unnecessary surgery on a child's genitals.[94]

Accordingly, the AAP's 2012 guidelines constitute an intentional scheme to revive Medicaid coverage in states that properly ended it, and thereby to defraud the federal and state Medicaid programs. In addition, under federal Medicaid law, state Medicaid agencies must conduct internal investigations of any report of fraud. They are required to refer suspected Medicaid fraud to the state's fraud control unit or "appropriate law enforcement agency,"[409] but they are not doing that either.

Proponents of genital cutting contend in their defense that it is preventive medicine; that ending Medicaid coverage is bad for health; that

---

405 Advisory Opinion of the Code of Ethics: Determining the Need for Medical or Surgical Intervention. *Am Academy of Ophthalmology.* 2016;1.
406 18 U.S.C. § 1347 (2012).
407 United States v. Bajoghli, 785 F.3d 957, 967 (4th Cir. 2015). <scholar.google.com/scholar_case?case=3630853056291459843>.
408 Circumcision Speaking Points (available from the author). 2012-08-27.
409 42 C.F.R. § 455.14–15 (2011).

the poor have a right to health parity; and that Florida's withdrawal of
Medicaid coverage for circumcision during the first year of a boy's life
resulted in a six-fold increase in medical costs for publicly funded circumcisions later in childhood. This is the age-old, untenable claim that
circumcision is good for health. Most boys in Europe, China, Japan, and
Central and South America are genitally intact and doing fine, and they
rarely need to be circumcised. Therefore, the costs to the Medicaid program in Florida did not increase six-fold because older boys needed to be
circumcised. Rather, once physicians in Florida were no longer allowed
to charge Medicaid for unnecessary circumcisions at birth, they circumcised older boys instead, which is more expensive as older boys can no
longer be physically restrained and they require general anesthetic. Regardless, because circumcision is unnecessary, it is not a covered Medicaid benefit.

FRAUDULENT DIAGNOSES AND MEDICAID FRAUD BY PHYSICIANS

The question arises, do physicians and hospitals also intentionally defraud the Medicaid program, like the American Academy of Pediatrics?
The answer in many cases is "yes".

Physicians falsely certify on the Medicaid billing form that the circumcision is medically necessary, when most are not. Since circumcision
is performed without a diagnosis, physicians also use a false diagnosis in
order to get paid. Physicians bill Medicaid using the billing code Z41:
"Encounter for procedures for purposes other than remedying health
state," the subsidiary billing code Z41.2, "Encounter for routine and ritual
male circumcision" in the absence of medical indication, and they use the
diagnosis group #795 for "Normal newborn."[410] The physicians are thereby admitting that they are circumcising healthy newborn boys routinely
or as a ritual in the absence of any medical indication or need,[2] which is
to say, without having a valid medical reason to perform the operation.
Physicians licensed to practice medicine should, and indeed they must
know, that "routine male circumcision," "ritual circumcision," meaning

---

410 ICD-10-CM Code Z41.2: Encounter for routine and ritual male circumcision. *ICD.Codes.*
   <icd.codes/icd10cm/Z412>.

performed for religious reasons, and "normal newborn" are not valid diagnoses, but those are the diagnoses that they use on the Medicaid billing form.

As in the past, physicians also often bill Medicaid for "phimosis" or a tight foreskin when a tight foreskin is normal in a newborn and until puberty. Even pathological phimosis, which is a medical condition, can usually be treated by stretching and applying topical corticosteroids.[410,411] Accordingly, the commonly used phimosis diagnosis is usually a scam. If the federal and state Medicaid agencies were complying with the law, and they reviewed even one payment for a neonatal circumcision, they would determine that it was not medically necessary.

Physicians who know that male genital cutting is not a covered benefit, but who bill Medicaid for it anyway, commit intentional Medicaid fraud, while the others are liable for recklessly violating Medicaid law.[412] (As discussed above, claims made with reckless indifference to their falsity meet the definition of fraud as well.)

CHAPTER SUMMARY

- Money fuels the multibillion dollar per year circumcision industry.
- Physicians are defrauding the Medicaid program by using false diagnoses and by falsely certifying that it is medically necessary to circumcise healthy boys.
- Under federal and state Medicaid law, the federal and state governments are not allowed to let physicians and their hospitals get away with this, but thirty-five states and the District of Columbia do.

---

411 Physicians also claim that circumcision is preventative medicine like vaccinations, but vaccinations are easily distinguishable. Unlike MGC, vaccinations do not involve the amputation of a body part; they are tested for safety; they are highly effective; and they are often the only way to prevent communicable diseases. MGC, by contrast, removes living tissue and a functional body part; it has a much higher complication rate, and it harms all boys and men; few males, if any, benefit from it; and any potential benefit can be achieved through other, less invasive, means. Boys, if given the option, would choose to be vaccinated against debilitating, untreatable diseases like polio, whereas boys communicate that they do not want to be circumcised, and men rarely volunteer to be. Moreover, people do not take to the streets to protest the fact that they have been vaccinated against dangerous communicable diseases, whereas they do protest having been circumcised.

412 NC Medicaid and Health Choice Clinical Coverage Policy No: 1A-22 § 3.2.2(a) (2015).

- In the face of declining Medicaid coverage, the American Academy of Pediatrics has engaged in a successful fraudulent scheme to revive and increase Medicaid coverage.
- Taxpayers have won the right to proceed on their claim in a Massachusetts lawsuit that the state is expending Medicaid funds unlawfully for unnecessary genital surgery.

Courts often observe that it is difficult to prove intent to defraud. A defendant can simply contend that he or she did not know that the claim was false or did not intend to deceive the plaintiff. Recognizing this, courts allow circumstantial evidence of intent to defraud. Given 150 years of unfair and deceptive conduct by the proponents of circumcision, and by the American Academy of Pediatrics since 1975, the evidence seems more than sufficient to prove intent to defraud by the AAP and by many, though not all, physicians who circumcise and their hospitals. For example, physicians must know that circumcision is painful and risky and that it removes erogenous tissue, but they are unlikely to disclose it. Using surprise and scare tactics and badgering parents all seem to be compelling evidence of acting bad faith.

Even if plaintiffs were unable to prove intent to defraud by a preponderance of the evidence, however, they have the claim that physicians, hospitals, and the AAP acted *recklessly,* without regard to the truth or falsity of their claims. When a physician acts with reckless indifference to safety, the plaintiff's claim for fraud still stands.

It seemed unfair though that infants and older boys below the age of consent would bear the burden of proving that they had been wronged. I began to think, who has the burden of proof in circumcision cases, the plaintiffs, here the boy and his parents, as is the norm in civil lawsuits, or the physician? It was only by chance that I recalled our torts professor telling us during the first semester of law school that because the physician-patient relationship is based on trust, physicians bear the burden of justifying every medical procedure, as discussed in Chapter 9 (Physicians Bear the Burden of Justifying Genital Cutting). Once a plaintiff claims that a physician did not have a valid reason to perform a procedure, *courts make the presumption that fraud has occurred.* The burden then falls on the physician to *rebut the presumption of fraud* by showing that he or she did have a valid medical reason to perform it.

United States case law shows that any breach of fiduciary duty or trust that causes damage constitutes so-called *constructive fraud.* Constructive fraud is also sometimes called *equitable fraud,* such as in New Jersey.

Under Roman law, if any law were unjust, it could be challenged. Similarly, in English courts, if a person lacked a claim in a court of law, he could seek justice in a court of equity. Now under English and U.S. law, courts of law and equity have merged, and there is a right to equitable relief for unfair and deceptive acts and practices.

Constructive fraud includes "all acts, omissions, and concealments involving breach of equitable or legal duty, trust or confidence, and resulting in damage to another."[412] For example, Georgia's statute provides, "Constructive fraud consists of any act of omission or commission, contrary to legal or equitable duty, trust, or confidence justly reposed, which is contrary to good conscience and operates to the injury of another."[413] Importantly, the California appeals court observed in *Salahutdin v. Valley of California, Inc.* in 1994, "Most acts by an agent in breach of his fiduciary duties [to the principal] constitute constructive fraud."[414]

When a fiduciary wins a vulnerable person's trust, and the plaintiff alleges that the defendant took unfair advantage of his position of trust to the detriment of the plaintiff, the presumption of fraud arises, *called constructive fraud.*[415] Where there is a breach of fiduciary duty, U.S. courts impute, infer, presume, or deem fraud to have occurred by operation of law. Constructive fraud is thus a legal fiction or construct. Importantly, a "fiduciary is liable to his principal for *constructive fraud* even though his conduct is not actually fraudulent"[414] (emphasis in original). That is, in a constructive fraud claim, the plaintiff does not need to prove intent to defraud. The purpose of the constructive fraud doctrine is to prevent the same unfair adverse consequences for the plaintiff as if the defendant had committed intentional fraud.[416]

In a Texas Court of Appeals case, *Crundwell v. Becker,* a patient suffering from abdominal pain testified that the physician had informed her that she had cancer when she did not, and that in reliance on that

---

413 GA. CODE ANN. § 23-2-51 (2010).
414 Salahutdin v. Valley of California, Inc., 24 Cal. App. 4th 555, 562 (1994).
   <scholar.google.com/scholar_case?case=68496945123275758 75>.
415 Terry v. Terry, 273 S.E. 2d 674, 677-79 (N.C. 1981), involving the sale of a business interest.
   <scholar.google.com/scholar_case?case=12733219259996420151>.
416 In re King Street Partnerships, 219 B.R. 848, 856 (B.A.P 9th Cir. 1998).
   <scholar.google.com/scholar_case?case=83253386693319365491>.

representation, she agreed to an unnecessary total hysterectomy (removal of her uterus). The patient's medical expert testified that there were less radical treatment alternatives to control her abdominal pain. On appeal, the court allowed her claim of constructive fraud to proceed to trial.[417]

U.S. case law substantiates that constructive fraud can arise from any of a multitude of unfair practices. These include a false statement that misleads the plaintiff such as a negligent misrepresentation,[418] and by extension a reckless misrepresentation; a material omission[419] or failure to disclose what a fiduciary knew or should have known;[420] unfair conduct such as self-dealing;[421] acting in bad faith, disloyally, consciously disregarding duties, or for personal gain;[422] taking advantage of a position of trust,[423] gaining an unfair advantage,[424] or obtaining a possible benefit.[424]

As documented in this book, physicians in the U.S. who circumcise healthy boys engage in every one of these unfair and deceptive practices. They all constitute a breach of fiduciary duty and constructive fraud. Since physicians will never be able to justify operating on a healthy child, they will never be able to defend against the claim that in soliciting, promoting, performing, and billing for genital cutting, they are committing constructive fraud.

417 Crundwell v. Becker, 981 S.W. 2d 880 (Tex. Ct. App. 1998). <scholar.google.com/scholar_case?case=13217238188300087187>.
418 Federal Land Bank Ass'n of Tyler v. Sloane, 825 S.W. 2d 439 (Tex. 1991). <scholar.google.com/scholar_case?case=17172414221833309328>.
419 Cantwell v. De La Garza, U.S. Dist. Court, WD Oklahoma (2018). <scholar.google.com/scholar_case?case=33112076777731126019>.
420 Karle v. Seder, 214 P.2d 684 (Wash. 1950). <scholar.google.com/scholar_case?case=7824574155812785213>.
421 Terry v. Terry, 273 S.E. 2d 674, 679 (N.C. 1981). <scholar.google.com/scholar_case?case=12733219259996420151>.
422 Ryan v. Gifford, 918 A.2d 341, 357 (Del. Ch. 2007) (stating that instances of bad faith include when "the fiduciary intentionally acts with a purpose other than that of advancing the best interests of the corporation, acts with the intent to violate applicable positive law, or where the fiduciary intentionally fails to act in the face of a known duty to act, demonstrating a conscious disregard for his duties.") <scholar.google.com/scholar_case?case=17080673641422634987>.
423 White v. Consolidated Planning, Inc., 603 S.E.2d 147, 156 (N.C. 2004). <scholar.google.com/scholar_case?case=26298824446929839251>.
424 Dawson v. Hummer, 649 N.E.2d 653, 661 (Ind. Ct. App. 1995). <scholar.google.com/scholar_case?case=13856981099867067611>.

- Importantly, plaintiffs in circumcision lawsuits do not need to prove intent to defraud or even that the physician was reckless because of the doctrine of constructive fraud.
- Once a plaintiff claims that a physician has breached the plaintiff's trust in the slightest way, a presumption of fraud arises. The burden then falls to the physicians to rebut the presumption of fraud by proving that the procedure was medically justified.
- Since circumcision is not medically indicated or justified, plaintiffs have claims against physicians and hospitals for constructive or equitable fraud.

26 Frivolous and Hence Fraudulent Defenses and Retaliation

Since unnecessary, non-consensual genital cutting is indefensible, what can physicians, hospitals, and state Medicaid offices do when they get sued? They can threaten the plaintiff or plaintiffs and raise frivolous defenses.

Retaliation

In a pending case in Ontario, Canada, for example, a young man sued the physician who circumcised him and Windsor Regional Hospital for battery (the circumcision was unlawful) and for negligence (the doctor performed the operation badly). The physician complained about being bothered in his presumably comfortable retirement, funded in part by having performed unnecessary circumcisions. Astonishingly, the physician and hospital then filed a counterclaim against the plaintiff's mother, claiming that if they were found liable, they would owe nothing: the mother would have to pay the damages because she had given written permission to have her son circumcised. If the operation were a battery as the plaintiff alleged, however, the physician is to blame for having offered it to the mother; and if he performed the operation negligently as alleged, he again is to blame and not the mother. The defendants' defenses are so lacking in merit that they seem designed to pressure the son to drop the lawsuit. He did not, and not surprisingly the relationship between the son and his mother has deteriorated.

In 2021, a man injured by circumcision and his parents sued the American Academy of Pediatrics for having issued fraudulent guidelines in 1989, based on Matthew Giannetti's 1999 law review article accusing the AAP of the same. The AAP's attorneys nonetheless claimed that the lawsuit is frivolous, and they demanded that the plaintiffs' lawyer dismiss all claims with prejudice. Otherwise, they said they would ask the court to sanction him as an attorney, which could result in disciplinary action, in theory the loss of his license to practice law, and to hold him liable for the

AAP's attorneys' fees and costs. The plaintiffs' attorney understood this to be a frivolous attempt to pressure him to drop the case.

Outspoken opponents of circumcision also risk being fired. Eric Clopper was terminated as a manager of a department at Harvard University after he put on an anti-circumcision play in the university's Sanders Theatre. His boss had approved every word and action in the play. In addition, Harvard's free speech manual encouraged free speech and promised to protect anyone in the community who engaged in it from retaliation. A leading psychologist opposed to circumcision in Australia lost his academic position for speaking out about it. A U.S. lawyer also lost his job after he suggested that his pregnant boss watch a video about circumcision. She claimed to have been offended by it, but on deposition she admitted that she had never watched it.

Thus, bad things can happen to the opponents of genital cutting when bad things should be happening to those who perform it, including being disciplined and subjected to criminal and civil penalties.

FRIVOLOUS DEFENSES

In the ongoing 2021 fraud suit against the American Academy of Pediatrics, the AAP argued that the suit should be dismissed because the plaintiffs' claim was for malpractice, not fraud. The AAP misunderstood the gravamen of the accusations against it. The claim is that the AAP used false claims and omissions to promote a procedure that physicians are not allowed to perform at all.

In the Massachusetts Medicaid case, discussed in Chapter 24 (Fraudulent Diagnoses and Medicaid Fraud), the plaintiffs' claims are straightforward: it is unlawful to use Medicaid to pay for circumcision because it is not medically necessary, and the state is neither requiring proof of medical necessity nor reviewing those payments as required. The state responded by appeals to authorities (e.g., physicians say that the circumcisions are medically necessary, and we presume they are right). Then the state used circular reasoning that circumcision is a covered benefit because we cover it. Next, it made the slippery slope argument that a ruling for the plaintiffs would open the floodgates to other lawsuits, as if it would be a bad thing to stop the state from paying for operations that people do not need, or a bad thing to force the state to review payments to ensure that they are medically necessary.

In the few circumcision lawsuits in the U.S. that I have seen or read about, the defendants advanced defenses that all seem frivolous to me. Since circumcision is so common in the United States, however, a judge would have to be extremely capable to see through these smoke screens.

CHAPTER SUMMARY

- When people object to circumcision or sue for damages, they may be subjected to threats and retaliation.
- In my opinion, defendants have raised frivolous defenses in circumcision lawsuits against them in the U.S.
- This brings to mind the Congressional testimony of tobacco industry chiefs in 1994 that cigarettes are not addictive. Two years later they were under investigation for possible perjury.

Chapter 27 shows how litigation considerations are largely favorable to the plaintiffs. Chapter 28 shows that nonetheless pitfalls abound in litigation generally and especially in circumcision litigation.

PLAINTIFFS

Circumcised boys and men are the principal plaintiffs of course. They have claims for battery (an unlawful touching), breach of fiduciary duty, and constructive fraud. They also have claims for intentional fraud, because when the physician defrauded their parents, the parents were acting as legal representatives of the boys. Thus, the boys and men were also deceived, as if the physicians had been talking directly to the boys instead of to their legal representative(s).

Parents also have battery claims, because the parents' permission was not fully informed, and claims for breach of fiduciary duty, constructive fraud, and for intentional fraud, as shown in this book. Parents can bring suit at any time during their son's minority, however, as legal representatives of their son.

DEFENDANTS

The defendants include the physician who performed the operation, of course. If the physician has died, his or her estate can be sued. The hospital can also be held liable under the doctrine of "respondeat superior" for the wrongful acts of the physician. Plaintiffs should therefore sue the physician and the hospital. Plaintiffs should seek to hold them jointly and severally liable, or each liable independently for all of the damages.[425]

Nurses who solicited parental consent and/or badgered the parent(s) can be sued as well. They must know that they should not be badgering parents. Nurses would not be held personally liable as they would prevail on a crossclaim against the attending physician and hospital. Another reason to sue nurses is that they might testify, as some say privately, that they do not want to assist with circumcisions and why, but their hospitals force them to do it.

---

425 Definition of "Respondeat Superior." <law.cornell.edu/wex/respondeat_superior>.

PHYSICIANS BEAR THE BURDON OF PROOF

As discussed in Chapter 11 (Remedies Under U.S. Civil Law), non-therapeutic male genital cutting is a prima facie or rebuttable case of a battery, a breach of fiduciary duty, and constructive fraud. Therefore, once a plaintiff asserts those claims (called "causes of action" in a lawsuit), the physician and the hospital bear the burden of justifying the operation. As argued, they will never be to justifying operating on a healthy child.

Plaintiffs, on the other hand, bear the burden of proving that the physician committed intentional fraud. They can prove this by circumstantial evidence. If not, they still have a fraud claim if they can prove that the physician acted with reckless indifference to the rights and health and safety of boys and the men they become.

MUCH EASIER THAN A MALPRACTICE SUIT

It is much easier for plaintiffs to bring a lawsuit for battery, breach of fiduciary duty, and constructive fraud than to bring a medical malpractice suit. Plaintiffs may need to meet preliminary requirements before bringing a malpractice suit, and in such suits the plaintiffs must have a medical expert, which is expensive. Circumcision lawsuits address "behaviors in which no physician should engage [and] regardless of the explanation given for that behavior ... [legal] consequences should flow."[164] Further, because "the plaintiff need only show that the physician's conduct violated basic rules of conduct regarding how all physicians are expected to act ... expert testimony may not be required."[164]

MUCH LONGER STATUTE OF LIMITATIONS

The statute of limitations sets a limit on how long a plaintiff is allowed to wait before suing. It is longer for fraud claims than for battery. For example,[426] a California court in the *Neilsens* case observed that the sta-

---

426 Neilsens v. Kazarian, (Cal: Ct. App. 2009). <scholar.google.com/scholar_case?case=824139701397092600>.

tute of limitations was two years for battery and intentional infliction of emotional distress, but three years for fraud and four years for breach of fiduciary duty.[427]

Importantly, the *Neilsens* court also held that the statute of limitations does not begin to run until the plaintiff discovers or has reason to discover the cause of action,[428] called the "discovery rule." Likewise, the New York Court of Appeals noted in *Simcuski v. Saeli,* "It is the rule that a defendant may be estopped to plead the Statute of Limitations where plaintiff was induced by fraud, misrepresentations or deception to refrain from filing a timely action."[429] In the current case against the American Academy of Pediatrics, the statute of limitations for the circumcised man had expired, but he and his parents invoked the discovery rule because they had only recently learned of the fraud. Circumcised boys, men, and their parents are likely to learn that they have been defrauded only upon reading this book. Therefore, that is when the statute of limitations begins to run. In addition, numerous states have implemented reforms extending the statute of limitation against the perpetrators of sexual abuse. Male genital cutting may well meet the definition of sexual abuse,[430] although it has not yet been prosecuted as such to date.

RIGHT TO WIN WITHOUT A TRIAL

When there are no legally relevant facts in dispute, there is no need for a jury to determine the facts, and a plaintiff is entitled to "summary judgment" or to win without a trial. Such cases can be decided "as a matter of

---

427 In Remis v. Fried et al., a New York court observed that the statute of limitations was three years for negligent misrepresentation, or the longer of six years from the wrongful conduct or two years from when the party knew or should have discovered intentional misrepresentation and fraud. Slip. Op. 50479(U) (N.Y. S. Ct. 2011). <scholar.google.com/scholar_case?case=1769601247657705237>.

428 WA Southwest 2, LLC v. First Am. Title Ins. Co., 240 Cal.App.4th 148, 156 (Cal. App. Ct. 2015). <scholar.google.com/scholar_case?case=16236181332745632586>.

429 Simcuski v. Saeli, 44 N.Y. 2d 442 (1978). <scholar.google.com/scholar_case?case=1634078491476144812>.

430 ChildUSA.org has compiled a summary of the civil and criminal statutes of limitations, if any, for child sexual abuse by U.S. state. See Summary of Child Sexual Abuse Statutes of Limitations (SOLs): Introduced, Signed into Law and State Laws by Category, CHILDUSA. <childusa.org/2019sol>.

law." The only material facts involving non-therapeutic male and female genital cutting are that the procedure is irreversible, harmful, unnecessary, and performed without the child's consent. In the German case in 2012, for example, the court ruled held without conducting a trial that circumcision is harmful and criminal assault. Likewise, in a United Kingdom case in 2016, the court ruled without a trial that boys have a right to decide the fate of the foreskin for themselves. There is no need for a trial in the U.S. either about whether circumcision is lawful or not. The plaintiff(s) will need to hire a medical expert or psychiatrist only to testify as to the amount of the damages.

DAMAGING PRIOR ADMISSIONS BY THE AAP

In litigation, the doctrine of equitable estoppel[431] may come into play. It is a "legal principle that prevents a person from asserting or denying something in court that contradicts what has already been established as the truth." In the past, physicians in the U.S. and their medical associations (the American Academy of Pediatrics, the American College of Obstetricians and Gynecologists, which endorsed the most recent 2012 AAP statement, and the American Medical Association) have made many admissions in writing that plaintiffs may be able to use to their advantage in lawsuits.

For example, in circumcision policy statements or guidelines between 1971 and 2012,[94,432,348] the American Academy of Pediatrics has stated correctly, and it has thereby admitted, that circumcision is not medically indicated (there is no need for it and it is not desirable);[373] that circumcision is a medically unnecessary non-therapeutic and elective procedure;[85,433] that "phimosis of the newborn" (a commonly used diagnosis) is not a valid medical indication for circumcision;[286] that the foreskin protects the glans for life and that any break in the foreskin affords an opportunity for infection;[433] that operators may not be well trained; that often no anesthetic is used, and that "local anesthesia adds an element of

431 Legal Dictionary. <dictionary.law.com/Default.aspx?selected=644>.
432 See generally American Academy of Pediatrics Circumcision Statements, Circumcision Information and Resource Pages, Statements. <cirp.org/library/statements/aap>.
433 1997 AAP Statement. <cirp.org/library/statements/aap/#a1997>.

risk";[85] that the "immediate hazards of circumcision of the newborn include local infection which may progress to septicemia, significant hemorrhage, and mutilation";[433] that the AAP does not know the incidence of complications;[94] that "[s]ome forms of FGC [female genital cutting] are less extensive than the newborn male circumcision";[434] that circumcision may reduce penile sensation and sexual satisfaction;[348] that circumcision cannot responsibly be viewed as protecting against sexually transmitted infection including HIV;[292] that "[a] program of education leading to continuing good personal hygiene would offer all the advantages of circumcision without the attendant surgical risk;"[292] that the benefits are not great enough to recommend it;[286] and that parents will need to take their own non-medical preferences into account. The American Medical Association stated in 1999 that circumcision is not medically justified; that "behavioral factors appear to be far more important than circumcision status" in causing sexually transmitted infections, including HIV; and that "circumcision cannot be responsibly viewed as 'protecting' against [sexually transmitted] infections."[94]

A CLASS ACTION LAWSUIT?

Some state consumer protection statutes provide that when an unfair and deceptive act or practice has injured numerous other similarly situated individuals, any injured person can bring a class action lawsuit on behalf of the class.[435] About 80% of males now living in the U.S., or roughly 132 million males, have been circumcised; the statute of limitations begins to run upon discovery of the fraud; circumcision is likely a $5 billion per year industry or larger; and it could be argued that the foreskin is priceless. Hence, plaintiffs' lawyers have a powerful financial incentive to bring a class action lawsuit in the United States. Class action lawyers

---

434 AAP Task Force on Circumcision. 1999 AAP Circumcision Policy Statement. See note #348.
("There are anecdotal reports (a) that penile sensation (b) and sexual satisfaction (c) are decreased for circumcised males.")
Link a: <archive.org/web/19991022030636/http://www.sexuallymutilatedchild.org/feelings.htm>;
Link b: <cirp.org/library/complications/money>;
Link c: <noharmm.org/bju.htm>.
435 Restatement (Second) of Torts § 908(2).

share a percentage of the damages awarded. A class action suit would be the quickest way to end the practice, and it would remove the serious obstacle of plaintiffs being unable to pay for litigation.

Insofar as it is a crime to circumcise a boy, it also seems to be a crime to manufacture any circumcision device such as a clamp. A medical expert stated at a Genital Autonomy conference that physicians cannot see how much foreskin is being pulled into the clamp. Thus, injuries to the glans or head of the penis are inevitable. Because these devices are unreasonably dangerous, manufacturers can be held strictly liable for them, meaning that the plaintiff does not need to prove that the manufacturer was negligent. Attorney David Llewellyn won a $11 million judgment when a Mogen clamp cut off part of the head of a boy's penis. The defendant had reportedly falsely claimed that injury was impossible with its use.[436] (The popular Gomco clamp's design also produces "a standardized, radically denuded organ, which has come to be widely regarded as the 'normal' condition of the U.S. penis."[325])

DAMAGES MAY BE LARGE, MULTIPLIED, AND UNINSURED

Damages May Be Large

Attorneys for the Rights of the Child has published a list of judgments and settlements involving genital cutting, the largest of which was $31 million.[437] Given that the foreskin is the most sensitive part of the penis, and men greatly value it (some might not part with it for any amount of money, and thus some view it as priceless), damage awards are likely to be large. As a battery is a tort, plaintiffs have the right to compensation for pain and suffering. In addition, faithless fiduciaries must make good the full amount of the loss that their breach has caused.[438] Plaintiffs who prevail on claims arising from breach of trust are also entitled to lost

---

436 Tagami T. Atlanta lawyer wins $11 million lawsuit for family, in botched circumcision. *Atlanta J Constitution.* 2010-07-19. <ajc.com/news/national/atlanta-lawyer-wins-million-lawsuit-for-family-botched-circumcision/P9Jewrh4v1GWStqGyfejiP>.
437 Attorneys for the Rights of the Child. Legal Victories. <arclaw.org/resources/legal-victories>
438 Prince v. Harting, 177 Cal. App. 2d 720 (Ca. Ct. App. 1960). <scholar.google.com/scholar_case?case=3693964523944007623>.

profits.[439] Plaintiffs are therefore also entitled to recover the surgeon's and hospital's profits from the operation, and if the hospital sold the foreskin to a pharmaceutical or cosmetics company, the profits from its unlawful resale as well.

Punitive Damages Should Be Awarded

Section 908 of the Restatement (Second) of Torts allows for an award of punitive damages. These are typically high for conduct that is "outrageous because of the defendant's evil motive or his reckless indifference to the rights of others." Interpreting that provision, a court in Pennsylvania ruled in 1970 that driving while intoxicated constitutes outrageous misconduct, given its obvious risks and the great probability of harm, regardless of the driver's person's motive or intent.[440] An Oregon court observed that where there has been a particularly aggravated disregard by a member of the medical profession of the professional duty to preserve life and health, punitive damages are appropriate, in part to deter such conduct.[441,442]

This book has shown that many physicians who circumcise and their hospitals and trade associations *do* have the unethical motive of enriching themselves at the expense of their patients. Regardless, it is outrageous to circumcise a healthy child: i it shows complete disregard for and reckless indifference to the child's health and rights. The United States Supreme Court has observed that punitive damages for wrongful conduct have long been a part of state tort law and that their purpose is compensation, punishment, and deterrence.[443] The Restatement (Second) of Torts § 908(2) provides that "[i]n assessing punitive damages, the trier of fact can

439 Id. "a faithless fiduciary must repay to the beneficiary of his fiduciary duties the entire profit that he has caused the beneficiary to lose."

440 Focht v. Rabada, 268 A.2d 157, 161 (Pa. Super. 1970). <scholar.google.com/scholar_case?case=97878524336688817719>.

441 Noe v. Kaiser Foundation Hosp., 435 P. 2d 306, 424-25 (Or. 1967). <scholar.google.com/scholar_case?case=15615901464990826593>.

442 Ghiardi JD. Punitive Damages in Wisconsin. *Marquette L Rev.* 1997 Spring;60(3):753-76. <scholarship.law.marquette.edu/cgi/viewcontent.cgi?article=2183&context=mulr>.

443 Pacific Mut. Life Ins. Co. v. Haslip et al., 499 U.S. 1 (1991). <scholar.google.com/scholar_case?case=17404474625320594258>.

properly consider the character of the defendant's act, the nature and extent of the harm to plaintiff that the defendant has caused or intended to cause and the wealth of the defendant."[444] Thus, courts can – and I suggest that they should – award punitive damages large enough to punish physicians and hospitals and to help end this practice without the need for more lawsuits.

Damage Awards May Be Uninsured

Finally, in *Cobbs v. Grant,* [211] the Supreme Court of California observed that physicians held liable for the intentional tort of battery might not be covered by malpractice insurance. Depending upon the state, physicians' insurance may not cover any of the claims discussed in this book. Malpractice insurers are insuring physicians and their hospitals against negligently performed operations, not against operations that the physicians should never have performed. Moreover, malpractice insurance contracts may expressly exclude fraud claims.[445] Physicians thus may be required to satisfy a judgment out of their personal assets. Physicians who cut healthy boys' genitals also risk jail time for criminal battery and for Medicaid fraud.

CHAPTER SUMMARY

- Litigation considerations are largely favorable to the plaintiff.
- Plaintiffs (boys, men, and parents as their legal representatives) have claims for battery, breach of fiduciary duty, and for constructive and intentional fraud.
- The statute of limitations for fraud begins upon discovery of the fraud, which likely will be upon reading this book. Therefore, in theory, any

---

444 The Massachusetts Consumer Protection Act, M.G.L. Ch. 93A § 9.
<malegislature.gov/laws/generallaws/parti/titlexv/chapter93a/section9>.
445 McCullough Campbell & Lane, LLP. Chart of Punitive Damages by State. The chart shows punitive damages by state and noting that punitive damages are insurable unless awarded for intentional misconduct.
<web.archive.org/web/20190304033741/https://www.mcandl.com/puni_chart.html>.

circumcised boy and man in the U.S. can bring suit for fraud, no matter how long ago he was circumcised.

- Circumcision suits are easier to bring than malpractice suits.
- Once plaintiffs bring their claims, physicians have the burden of rebutting the presumption that they are liable, but that will never be possible.
- Because it is self-evident that it is not medically necessary to amputate the foreskin of a healthy boy, the plaintiff has the right to prevail on "summary judgment," without expert medical testimony and without a trial (though a trial would be needed to prove damages).
- The American Academy of Pediatrics has made many admissions in the past that will be useful to plaintiffs in litigation and in making fraud claims.
- Damages may be large, multiplied, and uninsured.

The pitfalls for plaintiffs litigating any case are numerous.

In addition, no court in the United States has ever ruled that a physician is liable for a properly performed circumcision, even though physicians in the U.S. have circumcised more than one hundred million boys. The outcome of litigation is always uncertain, and even more so in circumcision cases.

Plaintiffs can become very emotionally involved with their lawsuit and be very unhappy if they lose. Litigation also proceeds at a glacial pace. The plaintiff(s) would need to engage in pre-trial discovery to prove that the physician made fraudulent misrepresentations or intentionally failed to disclose the truth about circumcision. Thus, plaintiffs could speed up the case a great deal by suing only for battery, breach of fiduciary duty, and constructive fraud, and moving for summary judgment without a trial on those counts. That way, they will win or lose quickly and inexpensively.

There is also bias in favor of the preserving the status quo. Judges who are circumcised themselves and especially religious adherents might be unconsciously biased in favor of the practice. For example, at a 2013 debate about the ethics and legality of circumcision, a Jewish professor spoke only once to say, "The bris [circumcision] is a beautiful ceremony!," leading Attorney Steven Svoboda to respond, "For whom?" Problematically, judges are unlikely to recuse themselves without being asked, but if a plaintiff does ask, the judge might become biased against the plaintiff.

Attorney Svoboda published an article in 2009, "A Treatise from the Trenches: Why Are Circumcision Lawsuits So Hard to Win?" He concluded,

> Barriers of many different types make successful circumcision-related lawsuits extremely difficult to bring. Actual cases we and others have brought show that among factors impeding progress are (1) financial risks; (2) procedural difficulties; (3) misconceptions and compassion misallocation among judges,

lawyers, jury members, the media, and the general public; (4) constraints unique to circumcision lawsuits that are imposed by statutes of limitation and statutes of repose; (5) need for parental participation in lawsuits; (6) problem of damages not being atrocious enough to justify litigation; and (7) the scarcity of helpful case law. … We will discuss the many reasons why potential plaintiffs never even make it to the filing stage. We will look at why judges and juries are starting to understand that just having a foreskin is not reason enough to have a circumcision.[446]

Public opinion is slowly turning against circumcision, however, and eventually the tide will turn in our courts as well. Meanwhile, while plaintiffs should hope to win, they should expect to lose.

CHAPTER SUMMARY

- Litigation is expensive and slow. Plaintiffs are unlikely to have the resources to bring their claims, while defendants have the resources to defend them. Plaintiffs can become very emotionally involved and be angry if they lose. Laws vary by state, and the theories in this book are untested and could be wrong. Plaintiffs must be prepared to lose.

---

446 Svoboda JS. A Treatise from the Trenches: Why Are Circumcision Lawsuits So Hard to Win? In: Denniston GC, Hodges FM, Milos MF, eds. *Circumcision and Human Rights.* 2009; pp.201-17). <researchgate.net/publication/225923940>.

PART VI:

WHAT CAN BE DONE TO END THIS SENSELESS VIOLENCE?

This Part discusses how hope springs eternal that the American medical profession will abandon this violent traditional practice, but that is unlikely to happen. It therefore recommends other possible actions, including litigation.

29 RECOMMENDATIONS

In 2012, the United Nations General Assembly announced an *Internatio-nal Day of Zero Tolerance for Female Genital Mutilation.*[447] Male and female genital cutting are analogous, and physicians are not allowed to discriminate on the basis of gender. There should be zero tolerance for male genital cutting as well worldwide. Instead, there is virtually 100% tolerance for it in the U.S. and among religious adherents in many other countries.

The argument has been made that banning circumcision would drive it underground among the religious, where it would be performed in un-sterile settings by individuals without medical qualifications.[448] It is not a defense to the enforcement of a law, however, that it conflicts with one's religious beliefs. The sons of the religious have the same right to an intact body and the right to decide its fate as every other boy and man, and they are entitled to the same protection from the risks and harms of genital cutting. Banning the practice would give religious adherents a powerful incentive to end the practice, whereas now they have none.

The industry is dying in the United States, but what can be done to speed its demise here, and to help end religious circumcisions?

HOPE SPRINGS ETERNAL, BUT LET'S BE REALISTIC

Physicians Who Circumcise

In an ideal world of zero tolerance, physicians who circumcise boys in the U.S. would join their counterparts in Europe in refusing to perform the operation and in condemning it. They would put down their knives and clamps and leave healthy boys' genitals alone. Some physicians in the U.S. such as Paul Fleiss[449] came to regret having performed it and

---

447 Link to article: <acslaw.org/inbrief/female-genital-mutilation-the-status-of-u-s-laws-restricting-the-practice>.

448 KNMG [Royal Dutch Medical Association]. Non-therapeutic circumcision of male minors. 2010; p. 5. <knmg.nl/circumcision>.

449 Fleiss PM. The Case Against Circumcision. *Mothering: The Magazine of Natural Family Living.* 1997 Winter; p. 36-45. <cirp.org/news/Mothering1997>.

stopped. Perhaps some physicians and nurses reading this book are realizing for the first time that they have been seriously harming boys and men, violating their rights, and exposing themselves to potentially uninsured liability every time they perform the operation.

But those who are still performing it, despite the increasing opposition to it, seem unlikely to stop. As Upton Sinclair wrote, "It is difficult to get a man to understand something when his salary depends upon his not understanding it." In court testimony, one physician stated that he had observed 5,000 circumcisions, and likely he had performed most of them. Although physicians who drop out are to be applauded, others will be standing by to circumcise the same boys.

American Medical Associations

The American Academy of Pediatrics, the American College of Obstetricians & Gynecologists, the American Academy of Family Physicians, and the American Medical Association should start over. They should convene neutral committees that include not only circumcised men but genitally intact men and women; the members of the AAP's committees on pain and on religion; physicians opposed to circumcision; ethical ethicists; legal scholars and human rights attorneys from around the world; and parents.

Regardless of the composition of the committees, these medical associations should all join The Royal Dutch Medical Association in condemning unnecessary genital cutting. But like The Tobacco Institute before it, the AAP is an apologist for this profitable industry, and it has gone dark in the face of withering criticisms of its 2012 guidelines, instead of using rational discourse to respond. The AAP also seems likely to remain silent in the face of the new research from Canada suggesting by association that circumcision does not reduce the risk of HIV, the centerpiece of the AAP's claims in 2012. It is a fraud for the AAP to promote circumcision to the public based on the claim that it reduces the risk of HIV, and then not to disclose that its claim has been proven false. Thus, U.S. medical associations seem very unlikely to change their pro-circumcision stance.

Hospitals

Hospitals should ban physicians from performing the procedure. But given how profitable circumcision is, and the fact that some hospitals sell the unlawfully harvested foreskins, which is likely very profitable, that seems unlikely to happen either.

Legislative Bans

The federal government and state legislators should pass gender neutral legislation banning unnecessary genital cutting. Proposed legislation to that effect has not passed even in Denmark and Iceland, however, where circumcision is virtually unknown and widely viewed as repugnant. There seems no chance of a national ban in the U.S. Moreover, a U.S. District Court ruled the federal female genital mutilation statute unconstitutional, as a matter that must be left to the states, so a federal ban on male genital cutting might be found unconstitutional as well.

A citizen's initiative in 2011 for citizens to vote on a circumcision ban in San Francisco did not make it out of the gate, despite the fact that citizens have a constitutional right to petition the government for redress. This is yet another example of how circumcision is *sui generis* or unlike anything else, and how when it comes to circumcision, those in authority ignore the rules. Physicians lobbied the state government, blocked the ballot initiative, and passed legislation falsely claiming that circumcision has an array of medical benefits.[450] When opponents of circumcision tried to pass legislation in Massachusetts banning circumcision, the Jewish chair of the committee vowed to her constituents that the bill would never leave her committee, and it did not. A newspaper article suggested that the proposed ban would pass "when pigs fly." Legislators are political animals, and to date they have bowed to pressure from physicians and religious advocates. Still, it is worth trying to persuade state legislators to propose a ban.

---

450 Gov. Brown Signs Bill to Prevent Male Circumcision Bans In California. *KPIX 5*. 2011-10-02. <sanfrancisco.cbslocal.com/2011/10/02/governor-brown-signs-bill-to-prevent-male-circumcision-bans-in-california>.

Medicaid

The U.S Centers for Medicare & Medicaid Services has a legal duty to announce to all states that it is unlawful for them to use Medicaid to pay for circumcision, except when it is medically necessary. It should call upon the states to require proof of necessity and establish institutional review boards to review payment, as required by federal and state law. But in the lawsuit in Massachusetts, the federal agency supported the state and steadfastly refuses to carry out its legal obligations.

The arguments against Medicaid coverage are so persuasive that hopefully some of the thirty-five states still paying for it will stop doing so. Paying for unnecessary surgery violates federal and state law; the operation seriously harms all boys and men; ending coverage would save the federal government and state governments several billion dollars per year; the money saved would pay for medical care that patients actually need; and taxpayers would no longer be forced to pay for cosmetic surgery that parents usually elect because they prefer the appearance of the circumcised penis.

WHAT ELSE CAN BE DONE (OTHER THAN LAWSUITS)

More Opposition by Physicians

Perhaps some physicians are opposed to circumcision but do it because hospitals pressure them to do so. These physicians have a duty to "just say no," and they could do so en masse.

It is likely that the obstetricians and pediatricians in the U.S. who do not perform the operation are opposed to the practice, since they would be paid to perform it. But they remain silent, likely out of deference to their colleagues who do. These physicians may not be aware that they are breaking the law too. They are required to report circumcision as child abuse,[451] to work to end it as it is unlawful and contrary to the best

---

451 AMA Code of Medical Ethics, Opinion 8.10. <ama-assn.org/delivering-care/ethics/preventing-identifying-treating-violence-abuse>.

interests of the patient,[452] and "to report physicians … engaging in fraud or deception, to appropriate entities."[191] It is an embarrassment to the American medical profession that European medical experts are taking the lead in opposing the practice in the United States.

Nurses Should Refuse to Participate En Masse

A nurse informed me that some nurses hate circumcision and think it is evil. "There are nurses who will not work day shifts on mothers because they refuse to assist with the circumcisions. My sister is an OB nurse, and she absolutely hates circumcisions as well. The problem is, some hospitals force the nurses to assist with circumcision."[453] It does not do any good for the boys, however, that these nurses do not like what they are doing to the boys. According to the American Nursing Association ethics committee, "Health care agencies [must] pay close attention to potential for human rights violations as they relate to patients, nurses, health care workers, and others within their institutions." Nurses are required, like physicians, to "always stress human rights protection and uphold the values and ethics of the profession." They must "advocate for human rights of patients." They are required to "examine the conflicts arising between their own personal and professional values and the values and interests of others who are also responsible for patient care and health care decisions, and they must address these conflicts in ways that ensure patient safety and promote the best interests of the patient."[454] In other words, nurses, like physicians, have a duty to "just say no" to genital cutting, as Marilyn Milos did. It crosses a line that no medical professional is allowed to cross. Nurses should tell those in authority that it is wrong, and that they are not allowed to participate in it. They have leverage too if they all threaten to quit en masse. It also would be very influential if the

---

452 AMA Code of Medical Ethics, Principle III. See note #191.

453 Personal communication. 2021-08-23.

454 ANA Center for Ethics and Human Rights. The Nurse's Role in Ethics and Human Rights: Protecting and Promoting Individual Worth, Dignity, and Human Rights in Practice Settings. Revised Position Statement. 2016.
<nursingworld.org/~4af078/globalassets/docs/ana/ethics/ethics-and-human-rights-protecting-and-promoting-final-formatted-20161130.pdf>.

American Nursing Association issued guidelines denouncing circumcision.

Regulate the Practice

A more promising route than trying to ban male genital cutting outright would be for states to begin to regulate it. Permission hidden in hospital forms, solicitation at the hospital, and badgering must be banned. Parents do not have the right to elect circumcision, but they certainly have the right to be fully informed. Unless states ban the practice, they should require a model consent form that tells parents the truth about the practice. Physicians and nurses should be required to make the same disclosures orally as well.

Private Insurance

As mentioned, a private insurer covered a surgery in my family only after determining that it was medically necessary. Private insurance companies are wasting a great deal of money and shortchanging their stockholders by paying for unnecessary and unlawful circumcisions.

More Education

The intactivist organizations mentioned in the Prologue have done a magnificent job educating the public. At the Genital Autonomy conference in 2011, I knew everyone there, and most were middle-aged or older. By 2019, there were so many participants, mostly young people, that even the founder of the movement, Marilyn Milos, did not know some of their names. This is encouraging for the future. Still, education is slow going when the U.S. circumcision industry promotes circumcision at every turn.

Videotaping the Sales Pitch

It would be very useful if, when asked *The Question,* parents turned on their smartphones. That would document when medical professionals solicit their permission, tell them nothing about the practice, hide the truth about it, or badger them. It would be useful to post these in a central place online to document how medical professionals are doing more selling then telling.

LAWSUITS

Fighting the circumcision industry, however, is like the game of whack a mole. Brian Earp, who writes extensively about ethical aspects of the practice, explains:

> There is a veritable truckload of bullshit in science. When I say bullshit, I mean arguments, data, publications, or even the official policies of scientific organizations that give every impression of being perfectly reasonable – of being well-supported by the highest quality of evidence, and so forth – but which don't hold up when you scrutinize the details. Bullshit has the veneer of truth-like plausibility. It looks good. It sounds right. But when you get right down to it, it stinks.
>
> In this story, Lord Voldemort is a prolific proponent of a certain controversial medical procedure, call it X, which many have argued is both risky and unethical. It is unclear whether Lord Voldemort has a financial stake in X, or some other potential conflict of interest. But in any event he is free to press his own opinion. The problem is that Lord Voldemort doesn't play fair. In fact, he is so intent on defending this hypothetical intervention that he will stop at nothing to flood the literature with arguments and data that appear to weigh decisively in its favor.
>
> … These letters are not typically peer-reviewed … instead, in most cases, they get a cursory once- over by an editor who is not a specialist in the area.
>
> So why doesn't somebody put a stop to all this? As a matter of fact, many have tried.
>
> A similar phenomenon can play out in debates in medicine. In the case of Lord Voldemort, the trick is to unleash so many

fallacies, misrepresentations of evidence, and other misleading or erroneous statements – at such a pace, and with such little regard for the norms of careful scholarship and/or charitable academic discourse – that your opponents, who do, perhaps, feel bound by such norms, and who have better things to do with their time than to write rebuttals to each of your papers, face a dilemma. Either they can ignore you, or they can put their own research priorities on hold to try to combat the worst of your offenses.

It's a lose-lose situation. Ignore you, and you win by default. Engage you, and you win like the pig in the proverb who enjoys hanging out in the mud.

… The amount of energy necessary to refute bullshit is an order of magnitude bigger than to produce it.[455]

It is certainly tiresome for opponents of circumcision to have to refute these never-ending false claims and omissions. In the opinion of George Denniston, President of *Doctors Opposing Circumcision,* and in mine, having seen how physicians and their trade associations use their best efforts to perpetuate circumcision at every turn, the only way to speed the demise of the industry is to bring lawsuits and to hold physicians and hospitals liable for the harm that they cause.

Circumcised Boys, Men, and Their Parents Can Bring Suit

This book therefore encourages circumcised boys, men, and their parents to sue physicians and hospitals, subject to the disclaimer near the end of this book, represented by lawyers. The more lawsuits, the better. That is the only way for boys and men to recover compensation for their losses. If you just learned about how the medical profession took unfair advantage of you or your son, hopefully you will not only get angry but will want to get justice and compensation. It also would be useful to raise a war chest to help finance these lawsuits.

---

455 Earp BD. The Unbearable Asymmetry of Bullshit. *Quilette.* 2016-02-15. <quillette.com/2016/02/15/the-unbearable-asymmetry-of-bullshit>.

If a class action lawsuit on behalf of all circumcised boys and men is possible, all injured parties could join the lawsuit at no cost to themselves. Given that most males in the U.S. are circumcised, the payoff for the attorneys if they prevail would be immense. This book provides a blueprint for those lawsuits.

How Courts Should Decide Circumcision Cases

Then everything will depend upon the courts. Courts in the U.S. often decide cases based on precedent. They should follow the lead of courts in Europe that have already considered this question numerous times, and that are reaching a consensus about how these cases should be decided: for boys, men, and their parents, and against physicians and religious adherents.

Courts should take judicial notice of the material or legally relevant facts, as have European courts, that circumcision is not medically indicated or medically necessary; that it is performed without the diagnosis of a medical condition requiring it; that it is harmful; that it is irreversible – it "changes the child's s body permanently and irreparably;" that it is performed without the child's consent, since minors are not of legal age; and that it is contrary to the best interests of the child.[232]

U.S. courts should rule without a trial, as the court did in Cologne, Germany in 2012, that circumcision for non- medical reasons violates the child's right to bodily integrity and self-determination, which supersedes the parents' rights, and constitutes criminal assault.[232] Courts should also rule that non-therapeutic circumcision is a battery, breach of fiduciary duty, and intentional and constructive fraud. What may happen is that some lower courts make erroneous rulings. Hopefully, courts of appeal will correct them, but that is by no means certain either.

In 1985, Wallerstein wrote, "routine newborn nonreligious circumcision will soon pass from the scene to join blood-letting and cupping in medical history."[89] Unfortunately, his prediction was premature as the American medical profession has doing everything possible in the interim to perpetuate the practice. Thus, although circumcision is a dying industry, it is dying very slowly. Absent lawsuits, and perhaps an avalanche of them, it may take many more decades before this barbaric ancient practice meets its inevitable end in the United States. Meanwhile, millions more defenseless boys and the men they become will be forcibly constrained, subjected to the great pain, risks, and physical and psychological harms of unnecessary genital cutting in violation of their most basic rights, and to the indignity of having the most intimate and sensitive part of their penis permanently removed, when there is no need or valid medical reason to do so, and when they would not choose to part with their foreskin if given the choice. Ending male circumcision by physicians in the U.S. will also take away from religious adherents the argument that it is good for health. Reducing male genital cutting may also reduce female genital cutting worldwide.

CHAPTER SUMMARY

- There should be the same zero tolerance for male genital cutting as there is for female genital cutting.
- The American medical profession has proven to be incapable of policing unnecessary surgery in general and unnecessary male genital surgery in particular.
- There is no hope of a legislative ban by the federal government or any U.S. state, and momentum has stopped among states ending Medicaid coverage. On the other hand, if legislation were passed legalizing circumcision, it would violate the inalienable rights of the child and be unconstitutional and invalid.
- Other than lawsuits, what can be done? Physicians in the U.S. have a duty to speak out against it. Nurses should refuse to participate en masse. The practice should be regulated. There should be bans against permission hidden in hospital forms, solicitation at the hospital, and badgering. Consent forms must fully inform parents about the risks and harms. More education is needed.
- Parents should also videotape and post online in a central place what medical professionals tell them about circumcision, if anything.

- Given that there is a veritable truckload of [B.S.] about circumcision, however, lawsuits are the only way to hasten the demise of the industry.

CONCLUSION

Because this book has covered a lot of ground, here is a summary of its contents, much like an abstract of an academic article.

The Prologue discussed how nurses or physicians in most hospitals in the United States surprise parents by asking them, shortly after boys are born whether they want to have their son circumcised or not *("The Question")*. Half the time, the nurses or physicians do not tell parents anything about what they are offering. When they do *("The Talk")*, they are likely to invoke the 2012 guidelines of the American Academy of Pediatrics as an authority, and to tell the parents, in part, that they have the right to elect to have their son circumcised so that their son's penis will look like the father's penis. That false claim led to the question of whether the American medical profession is telling the truth and the whole truth about the practice.

Chapter 2 outlined "the debate" between the proponents of genital integrity and the proponents of genital cutting. The book's thesis is that it is indefensible to cut off a healthy part of a child's body. It will never be possible for physicians to justify it. The arguments in favor of it are all pretextual and designed to sell it to unsuspecting parents representing their sons.

Part I asked, what are the facts? Chapter 3 showed that the prepuce is an essential component of perfect health and very good for health. Chapter 4 showed that genital cutting is very bad for health. Chapter 5 showed that most boys would choose not to be circumcised if given the choice and able to make it.

Part II asked, what are the rights and duties of the parties? Chapter 6 showed that boys and the men they become have the right to bodily integrity, self-determination or autonomy and privacy, freedom of religion, and Equal Protection of the Law. Chapter 7 showed that genital cutting violates those rights of the child. Hence, physicians are not allowed to perform the operation, except in rare circumstances when it is medically necessary. Chapter 8 showed that parents also must respect the rights of the child, and that they do not have the right to elect to have their son circumcised except when it is medically necessary. Parents do, however, have the right to be told the whole truth about the procedure.

Part III asked, what legal remedies do circumcised boys, men, and their parents have? Chapter 9 showed that physicians have the burden of justifying unnecessary genital cutting without consent, but that will never be possible. Chapter 10 showed that circumcision is a crime – child abuse, criminal assault, and manslaughter when it is fatal – and in fact the perfect crime as it has never been prosecuted in the United States. The implication is profound, namely that all contracts involving circumcision are legally invalid and void. Chapter 11 showed that boys, men, and their parents have civil claims against physicians and hospitals for battery and breach of fiduciary duty. Chapter 12 showed how European courts are reaching a consensus that non-therapeutic circumcision is irreversible and harmful; that it violates a boy's right to personal security and self-determination, which supersedes the parents' religious and other rights; that it is a crime and unlawful; and that it is in the best interests of healthy boys to let them reach adulthood genitally intact, when they can decide whether they want to be circumcised or not (invariably not). Chapter 13 showed that although no U.S. court has ever held a physician liable for a properly performed circumcision, U.S. courts have not recognized an absolute parental religious right to circumcise boys either. Judges in the U.S., especially those who are religious adherents and men, may be unconsciously biased in favor of circumcision for religious and cultural reasons.

Part IV, the heart of the book, showed how circumcision is a fraud. Chapter 14 discussed how the past is prelude to the present. Physicians popularized genital cutting by appealing to Americans' puritanical instincts ("prevents masturbation"); by making frivolous claims such as that the foreskin is dirty and a source of disease; by making false medical claims that its removal prevents or cures more than one hundred diseases, including whatever was the disease of the day; by using false diagnoses like "long foreskin" and "tight foreskin"; and by unlawfully circumcising boys in the hospital without parental permission. Chapter 15 showed how American medical-trade associations and physicians have undisclosed multibillion dollar per year financial, religious, cultural, and personal conflicts of interest and biases in favor of perpetuating the practice. Chapter 16 showed that to prevail in a lawsuit alleging intentional fraud, a plaintiff must prove by direct or circumstantial evidence that he or she was intentionally deceived, or that the defendant acted in reckless disregard of the truth, and that as a result the plaintiff lost something of value and/or that the plaintiff had the legal right to keep. Chapter 17 showed how hospitals and private practices use *fraudulent advertising and marketing.* Chapter 18 showed how physicians and nurses engage in *fraudulent conduct* in the hospital. This includes targeting boys unable to object; targeting mothers who have just given birth, often on medications, and whom it can be presumed are legally incapacitated; using the high-pressure sales tactic of giving the parents only minutes to decide without benefit of a second opinion; and badgering parents until they agree to have their son circumcised. Chapter 19 discussed some of the many frivolous and *fraudulent reasons* that medical professionals advance to sell circumcision to parents, such as the claim that the circumcised penis is cleaner and will prevent a boy from being embarrassed in the locker room. Chapter 20 discussed the *fraudulent medical claim that circumcision is not harmful.* In fact, it risks many complications, physical and psychological, and it is sometimes fatal; and as it is painful and removes the most sensitive part of the penis, and destroys how the penis normally functions, it seriously harms all boys and men even when it is properly performed. Chapter 21 discussed the *fraudulent medical claim that circumcision is good for health.* It has little prospect of benefiting any boy or man, which violates the ethical obligation to perform a procedure on a child only when it will benefit the child. The only claimed benefit in childhood is a 1% reduction in urinary tract infections, but UTIs can be treated easily with antibiotics. Boys are not at risk of adult diseases, so adult diseases are irrelevant. In addition, even if circumcision slightly reduces the risk of penile cancer and some sexually transmitted diseases including HIV, which is unproven, those diseases can be prevented safely and much more easily and effectively without loss of the foreskin. Accordingly, there is no valid medical reason to circumcise a healthy boy. Chapter 22 showed how the American medical profession makes *fraudulent legal claims:* that physicians have the right to perform the operation;

that parents have the right to elect it; and that physicians are allowed to take orders from parents to operate on a healthy child. These big lies – that circumcision is good and not bad for health and that parents have the right to elect it – have perpetuated circumcision to the present day. Chapter 23 showed how physicians and hospitals use *fraudulent consent forms* to persuade parents to say "yes." Chapter 24 showed how physicians use *fraudulent diagnoses* like "newborn boy" and "phimosis" or a tight foreskin, an age-old scam, to get paid. They also commit *Medicaid fraud* by falsely claiming on Medicaid reimbursement forms that it is medically necessary to circumcise a healthy boy and by using false diagnoses. Chapter 25 showed how circumcision constitutes *constructive or equitable fraud,* even if intent to defraud is lacking. Chapter 26 showed defendants in circumcision lawsuits assert frivolous and hence *fraudulent defenses.*

In short, circumcision is a complex 150-year-old multibillion dollar per year scam, a hoax, a fraud.

Part V discussed litigation considerations. Chapter 27 showed that these are largely favorable to the plaintiffs. In many states, the statute of limitations for fraud begins upon discovery of the fraud. Plaintiffs have the right to prevail without a trial on their claims for battery, breach of fiduciary duty, and constructive fraud, as there are no facts in dispute and no possible defenses to those claims. Damages for severe pain and suffering and for the loss of most sensitive part of the penis for life, should be large. Physicians' insurance for malpractice or for a badly performed operation may not cover claims for unnecessary surgery and fraud. Chapter 28 showed that pitfalls abound in litigation, however, including the fact that U.S. courts have never held a physician liable for a properly performed circumcision; deeply rooted cultural bias in favor of the practice; and the fact that the industry has its back against the wall and is well financed. By contrast, plaintiffs often are unable to afford the high cost of lawyers and litigation. Plaintiffs should of course hope to win but they should expect to lose.

Part VI contained recommendations. Chapter 29 argued that genital cutting is such a bad thing that there should be zero tolerance for it, regardless of gender. Ending male genital cutting by physicians – taking away the argument that it is good for health – also may help to reduce male and female genital cutting worldwide for religious reasons. After 150 years of performing circumcisions and defending the practice, however, physicians and their trade associations have made clear that they are not going to stop circumcising boys until someone forces them to stop. The book therefore encourages lawsuits represented by counsel to obtain compensation and to deter the practice, subject to the legal disclaimer below.

To summarize the book, the verdict about the circumcision debate is as follows:

	THE FORESKIN	GENITAL CUTTING	WHO DECIDES?	ETHICAL AND LAWFUL?	VERDICT?
OPPONENTS	Good for health and valuable	Bad for health	The owner of the penis	No	All true
PROPONENTS	Bad for health and has no value	Good for health	His parents	Yes	All false

In short, courts should decide every circumcision case in favor of boys, men, and their parents, and against physicians, hospitals, and their trade associations.

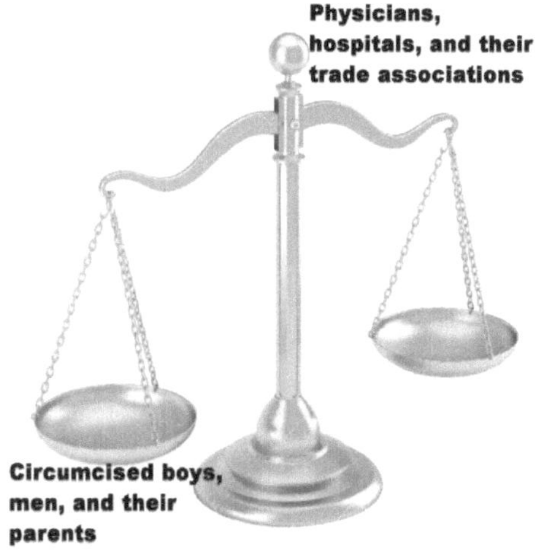

This book can also be summarized by reference to the optical illusion below. Do you see an attractive and let us assume a good young lady, or an unattractive and let us assume a bad old woman? Let us call former a good thing and the latter a bad thing.

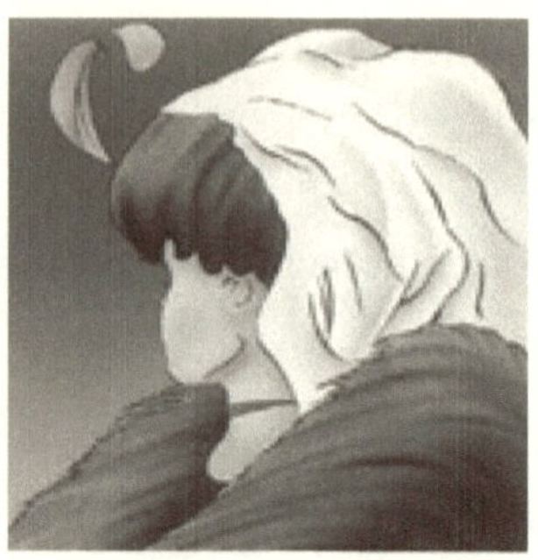

Physicians, their medical associations, and hospitals in the United States have spent the past 150 years successfully persuading the American public and the parents of newborn and older boys that they are good – you can trust them – and that circumcision is a good thing and indeed a very good thing. But the truth is that no one can trust anything that physicians who circumcise healthy boys and their trade associations claim in favor of it, and it is a bad and indeed a very bad thing: it causes immense suffering in the U.S. and worldwide. Regardless, it violates fundamental and inalienable rights of the child. In the circumcision-happy United States, it may be difficult for some to see this, but increasing numbers of lay people here, especially young people, are finally seeing it. Once you see it too, it will be impossible for you to unsee it.

EPILOGUE

Looking back on that day long ago when the Harvard physician pitched circumcision to me, I realized why I had been uncomfortable. First, I knew nothing about circumcision and had no choice but to trust the physician. Second, he pressured me by suggesting one invalid reason after another why I might or should elect it. Third, he expressly told me that circumcision is not medically justified, yet here he was offering to cut off part of my son's penis.

I feel that I dodged a bullet aimed at my son and that I was lucky to do so. Ironically, I had to learn the truth about the practice from the opponents of it, many of whom are not physicians.

Every hour of every day around the country, nurses and physicians are putting on a full-court press, targeting helpless infants and mothers who have just given birth, and using false claims, scare tactics, and relentless badgering to sell circumcision to unsuspecting and trusting young parents. No wonder the parents say "yes" a little more than half of the time, resulting in about 1.5 million circumcisions every year in the U.S. Meanwhile, undisclosed to the parents, physicians in most countries around the world are leaving boys' foreskins alone, those boys and the men they become are doing just fine, and they consider the foreskin of their penis to be of great value.

As an example of that, our son Geoffrey is thirty-four years old as of this writing. He has never suffered from any penile problem, and if he had, the problem could have been treated without loss of the foreskin. Like other genitally intact men, he considers it to be to his advantage to have one. I do not need to ask him whether he has ever thought to himself that it might be a good idea to check into a hospital and ask to have it cut off.

If I had a "do over" and knew then what I know now, I would have told the physician: my wife is "out of it," you are hiding the truth about circumcision, and it is unethical, unlawful, and indeed evil to cut off a healthy part of a child's body. You are enriching yourself at the expense of a helpless infant who is trusting you. I also would have put a waistband or ankle bracelet on my son saying, "Do NOT Circumcise, Do NOT Retract."[456]

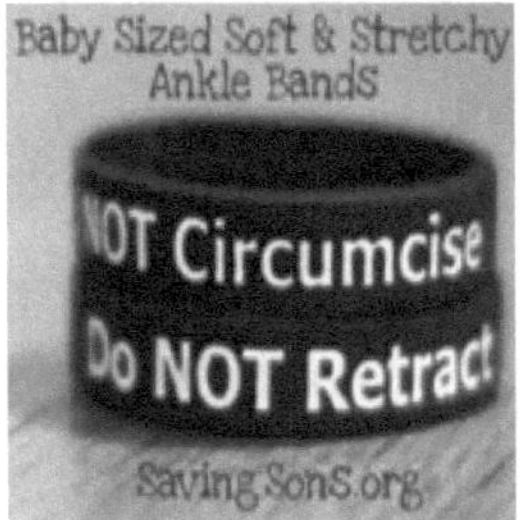

---

456 Available here: <etsy.com/listing/502616895/do-not-retract-do-not-circumcise-intact>.

And I would have taken my son out of the hospital at the first opportunity, because physicians are so enthusiastic about circumcising newborn boys that they have been known to take them out of the intensive care unit to do it.

When my son became a young man, I told him that the doctor had tried to sell circumcision to me. Actually, I told him, "When you were born, a doctor came for the foreskin of your penis – your mother was out of it – and I said no." He said, "Thanks, Dad" but he added, "it's not rocket science." More recently, this year, he said, "Who would cut off part of a baby's penis? What the fuck?" This comports with the comment by a European pediatrician that circumcision and setting up a task force to try to justify it is insane.[370] That is how many Europeans view it.

If you have a son, please do not welcome him into the world with probes, clamps, and knives. Just say "no." Your son will thank you; you will never regret it; and you will be helping to end this vicious thousands of years old cycle of unnecessary male, female, and intersex genital cutting.

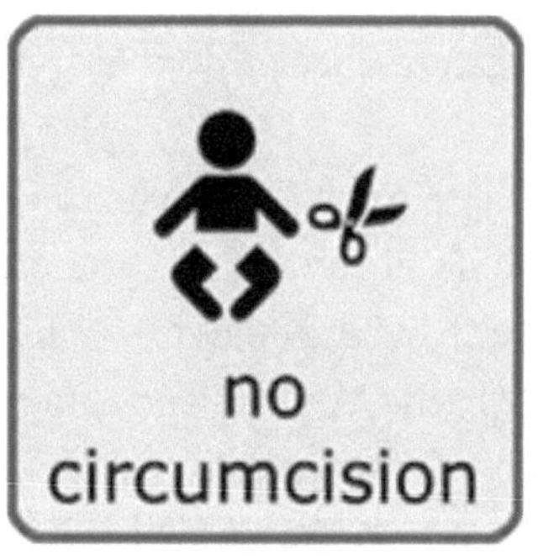

I certainly believe every word in this book to be true. It is based on simple facts and fundamental rules of medical ethics and law, as set out in a law review article in 2020 in the *Cornell Journal of Law and Public Policy.*[3] In addition, lawyers have sued the American Academy of Pediatrics for having issued fraudulent circumcision guidelines in 1989. In doing so, those lawyers are certifying that, to the best of their knowledge, they have valid claims. European courts are ruling in favor of boys and men, not their parents and physicians.

That having been said, the opinions and conclusions expressed in this book are mine and mine alone.

As courts have observed, it is also difficult to prove intent to defraud. I do not know what the members of American medical associations or individual physicians are actually thinking. Therefore, I am alleging that the most recent 2012 circumcision guidelines of the American Academy of Pediatrics are fraudulent, and that some (not all) physicians are defrauding parents, based on circumstantial evidence. Granted, some physicians and nurses are acting in good faith. Medical students who have never seen a circumcision before may not know that it is painful. Thus, individual physicians may not have committed intentional fraud. But once physicians have seen or performed a single circumcision, they know, but they usually fail in their duty to disclose it.

I also recognize that many people worldwide believe sincerely that circumcision is a religious requirement or tradition, and they are entitled to that belief. I recognize that many of them are not open to discussion. As discussed in Chapter 12 (European Cases), however, European courts have ruled that parents do not have the right to circumcise their son for religious reasons.

As a further disclaimer, I have written this book in my capacity as a legal scholar, and not as a practicing lawyer representing anyone. **I DO NOT REPRESENT THE READER OR ANY READER WHO BECOMES A PLAINTIFF IN A LAWSUIT. YOU COULD LOSE THE LAWSUIT AND SHOULD EXPECT TO LOSE IT. YOU ALSO WILL NEED TO HIRE YOUR OWN LAWYER** to represent you, and to ascertain independently whether you have a valid basis to bring suit in your state, and a reasonable prospect of prevailing. **NO LAWYER CAN GUARANTEE A FAVORABLE OUTCOME.** And as discussed, there are many pitfalls to any litigation, including that it is expensive.

Finally, I welcome respectful dialogue about this book, and will be glad to correct any errors brought to my attention.

ACKNOWLEDGMENTS

When reading books, I have often been surprised by the number of people authors thank in their acknowledgments. Now I understand! I am immensely grateful to the many people who taught me, inspired me, and supported me while I wrote this book.

Foremost I thank my wife and physician **Gail** as she has been my sounding board during the no doubt seemingly endless seven years that it took to think through and write the law review article on which this book is based and then to turn the article into this book. During our discussions, she often did helpful research into the medical literature. I really cannot thank my wife enough for her knowledge, help, patience, and encouragement. She is not responsible for any content in the book, of course.

I am grateful that our son **Geoffrey** allowed me to discuss his genitally intact status in the book. He has been very supportive of this project and indeed of everything that I do. My daughters **Carolyn** and **Christy** have been very supportive of my writing the book as well.

I am indebted to **Robert Van Howe,** my gifted former law student, **Felix Daase** from Germany, now a law student in Germany, and **Travis Wisdom,** for co-authoring the fraud article published in a Cornell law journal on which this book is based.

Three of my students proofread this book, and I thank each of them for their hard and valuable work. These include **Tyler White,** now a law student at Boston College law, and two other law students of mine, **Katlyn Santo** and **Lauren Foley,** who both plan to go to law school as well.

Thanks goes to **Petrina Fadel** of *Catholics Against Circumcision.* She researched the states that have ended Medicaid coverage, made other valuable contributions to the book, and proofread it on short notice as well.

I hold **Marilyn Milos, Robert Van Howe,** and **Steven Svoboda** in the highest esteem as founders, leaders, and creative luminaries in the fight against unnecessary genital cutting, and as my teachers and mentors. They each deserve a Nobel Prize for having worked so hard and sacrificed so much to end the needless suffering caused by this practice.

I also have the highest regard for the brilliant and prolific young ethicist **Brian Earp,** who burst upon the scene with a profusion of novel and persuasive ideas about this topic. Thank you, Brian, for your comments on my articles and this book. I look forward to reading and learning from whatever you write.

My admiration goes to **Georganne Chapin** for her inspiring leadership of *Intact America,* and to **Eric Clopper** for his fearless advocacy against religious circumcision.

I have met so many wonderful and inspiring people at the *Genital Autonomy* conferences. One was **Holm Putzke,** the law professor whose legal scholarship laid the foundation for the ruling in Cologne, Germany that it is a crime for physicians to circumcise boys for religious reasons.

Ronald Goldman is a leading scholar about the psychological harm that circumcision causes.

Thanks go to **Tim Hammond** for leading two surveys of men harmed by circumcision, and for his effort to raise a war chest to help finance lawsuits.

I also have great admiration for **Brother K** and for the men and women in **The Bloodstained Men** who take to the streets to protest genital cutting.

David Llewellyn, a fellow UVA law alumnus, the leading circumcision trial lawyer in the country, is very impressive. I thank David for using his many years of experience to sue the American Academy of Pediatrics for having issued fraudulent guidelines in 1989.

It has been a great pleasure as well to work on three circumcision cases with Attorney **Andrew DeLaney** of New Jersey. Andrew is a fearless and zealous advocate for his clients, and a very persuasive orator. It bodes well that such a young and capable attorney is developing a law practice in intactivist litigation.

Special thanks go to three members of *Doctors Opposing Circumcision:* **George Hill,** who wrote the Foreword for this book; attorney **John Geisheker,** who reviewed the legal arguments in it; and DOC's president, **George Denniston,** who believes that litigation is the only way to end circumcision quickly.

Finally, thank you to **Ling Zeng** for designing the cover, to **Chris Green** for helping publish the 1st edition of the book, and to **Ulf Dunkel,** a professional book editor, for editing and formatting this second edition.

In fact, thanks to every person anywhere in the world who is working to end unnecessary male, female, and intersex genital cutting!

In unity for the children,

Peter W. Adler

Wellesley, Massachusetts
January 15, 2022

Revised July 28, 2022

Peter W. Adler was born in England, but grew up in the United States, and he is a dual U.S.-U.K. citizen. He earned a B. A. in Philosophy from Dartmouth College (magna cum laude and Phi Beta Kappa); a M. A. degree in Philosophy and Ethics from Cambridge University (with Honours); and a J. D. degree from the University of 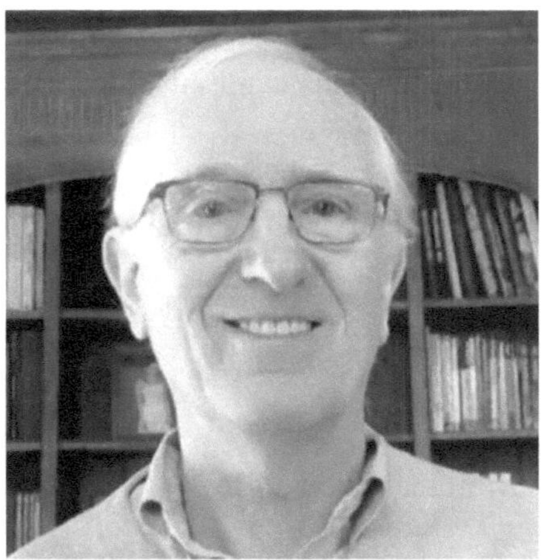 Virginia School of Law, where he was an editor of the *Virginia Law Review* and the *Virginia Journal of International Law.*

From 1983 to 1996, he practiced civil litigation and corporate law in the Boston area and became a name partner at a law firm in charge of civil litigation.

He left the practice of law in 1996 to start one of the first ecommerce businesses. He sold it to a Fortune 500 company in 1999, where he helped to build and run its ecommerce department. He ran another ecommerce company from 2002 to 2015.

Since 2015, he has taught International Law, Business Law, and International Business at the University of Massachusetts, and he leads the Study Abroad program to Copenhagen. In 2019 he won an award for Excellence in Teaching.

Professor Adler has published ten law review articles about circumcision and the law, two of which have provided the foundation for pending lawsuits. He is also active in circumcision litigation.

He lives with his wife Gail in Wellesley, Massachusetts. They have three children and three grandchildren. He enjoys tennis, bicycling, and sailing and kayaking on Cape Cod.

APPENDIX – AFFIDAVIT OF ROBERT VAN HOWE, M.D.

[Robert Van Howe M.D. submitted this affidavit under penalties of perjury in the Massachusetts Medicaid case discussed in this book. As he states in Paragraph 4, "Non-therapeutic circumcision or genital cutting falls outside the scope of medical practice worldwide and in the United States."]

***

I, Robert S. Van Howe, M.D., M.S., being duly sworn, do attest and affirm the following:

1. I am a physician and pediatrician licensed in the states of Michigan and Wisconsin. I was the founding Chief and Professor of the Department of Pediatrics at the Central Michigan University College of Medicine, and I currently hold the position of Clinical Professor in the Department of Pediatrics and Human Development at the Michigan State University College of Human Medicine.

    Education: I hold an M.D. degree from the Loyola University Stritch School of Medicine, completed a Pediatrics residency at Children's Hospital of Wisconsin, and have a Master of Science degree in Clinical Research Design and Statistical Analysis from the University of Michigan School of Public Health. I am Board Certified in Pediatrics through the American Board of Pediatrics.

    Publications: I have authored at least sixty-nine scientific articles and letters on the topic of infant and child circumcision that have been published or are scheduled to be published in peer-reviewed medicolegal journals including Pediatrics, the in-house journal of the American Academy of Pediatrics, the highly ranked *Journal of Law, Medicine & Ethics,* and the *Cornell Journal of Law and Public Policy.* I have also authored several book chapters and have lectured internationally about infant and child circumcision.

Peer-Reviewer: I have been a peer reviewer for the following medical journals and publishers: *American Journal of Public Health, Annals of Family Medicine, Archives of Disease in Children, Archives of Pediatrics & Adolescent Medicine, BMC Oral Health, BMC Public Health, BMC Urology, British Journal of Urology, The Cochrane Renal Group, European Journal of Obstetrics & Gynecology and Reproductive Biology, International Journal of Cancer, International Journal of Gynecology & Obstetrics, International Journal of STD & AIDS, Journal of Pediatrics, Journal of Public Health in Africa, The Lancet, Lancet Infectious Diseases, Pediatric Dermatology, Pediatrics, Sexually Transmitted Infections, Southern Medical Journal, Springer Publications, THYMOS: Journal of Boyhood Studies,* and *Yale University Press.*

Expert Opinion: I have been invited to provide my expert opinion on the subject of infant and child circumcision by the American Academy of Pediatrics (AAP), the U.S. Centers for Disease Control and Prevention (CDC), and the World Health Organization (WHO).

Awards: I have won several awards for excellence in research and teaching.

My contact information is available upon request through the attorneys in this matter.

2. I declare as follows, and I give my professional medical opinion here without any equivocation or hesitation. I have kept references to the medicolegal literature to the minimum to save space in this filing with the court, but I can provide a comprehensive list upon request.

3. Elective, non-therapeutic male circumcision (ENTMC), usually performed at or near birth but sometimes later in childhood, is an unnecessary and irreversible invasive genital procedure.

4. Without the need for treatment, the physician's and surgeon's certificate, evidencing a license to practice medicine, does not authorize the holder to use drugs or to use devices to sever or penetrate the tissues of the genitals of normal newborn males. Physicians in the United States are outliers among physicians worldwide in circumcising healthy boys, and they fail to meet universal professionally recognized standards of health care. Non-therapeutic circumcision or genital cutting falls outside the scope of medical practice worldwide and in the United States.

5. Newborn male circumcision is not recommended by a single national medical organization in the world including the United States. Several national and international medical organizations recommend against the procedure, citing the lack of medical evidence to support the practice and ethical and human rights concerns.

6. Non-therapeutic circumcision began as a sacrificial religious ritual, a painful rite of passage, and to suppress sexuality. Physicians introduced it to the United States in the late 1800s to early 1900s to prevent masturbation, then considered a cause of illness. Physicians claimed under medical theories circulating at the time that circumcision cured or prevented more than 100 diseases. These theories were subsequently replaced with the germ theory of disease, but as a result circumcision became a deeply embedded cultural norm in the United States, so the practice is self-perpetuating.

7. Parents in the United States who elect to have their son circumcised, after physicians or nurses under their direction solicit their permission, usually do so for cultural reasons, based on the parents' own religious, cultural, and personal aesthetic preferences – for example, the preference when the father is circumcised for the son's penis to "look like" the father's penis – rather than for medical reasons. In accordance with professional ethical standards, physicians are forbidden from acquiescing to parental requests to perform unnecessary medical procedures on their children.

8. Eighteen states in the United States ended Medicaid coverage of infant and child male circumcision, because it is not medically necessary and/or because they considered it a poor use of scarce Medicaid resources.

9. Physicians who circumcise healthy boys are engaging in a pattern of performing unnecessary surgery.

PAIN, RISKS, AND HARM

10. Unnecessary surgery is painful; it risks many minor and serious complications, including death; it removes healthy tissue and a functional body part, leaves a scar as evidence of a wound; and it can cause psychological harm. The same is true of ENTMC.

11. ENTMC is one of the most painful procedures in neonatal medicine. Often no anesthesia is used, and anesthesia is not completely effective.

12. Newborn male circumcision carries many minor and serious risks. Procedures without a medical indication that carry any risk of a complication and that are undertaken without the valid consent of the patient, or in the case of ENTMC the healthy person, are not within the scope of medical practice.

13. Newborn male circumcision carries the risks (ranging from 2% to 35%) of:[A1]
    (a) interrupting infant feeding, especially breastfeeding
    (b) disrupting the baby's sleep pattern for up to one week following the procedure
    (c) invoking behavioral changes
        i.   changes in initial maternal-infant bonding
        ii. crying longer and louder when receiving vaccinations at 4 and 6 months of age

iii. autism

iv. attention deficit disorder

v. engaging in different sexual practices than males not circumcised

(d) an overall increase in sexually transmitted diseases (gonorrhea, Chlamydia, non-specific urethritis)

(e) bleeding (heavy bleeding in about 2% to 9%, resulting in shock, the need for blood transfusions, or death)

(f) infections (1% to 5% of infants) – localized or systemic infections including:

i. bacteremia

ii. septicemia

iii. meningitis

iv. osteomyelitis septic hip arthritis

v. lung abscess

vi. staphylococcal scalded skin syndrome

vii. gangrene of the penis and scrotum

viii. scrotal abscess

ix. impetigo

x. erysipelas

xi. necrotizing fasciitis of the abdominal wall (gangrene)

xii. tetanus

xiii. herpes simplex infection

xiv. methicillin-resistant Staphylococcus aureus (MRSA) infections (12 times more common in circumcised male infants)

(g) necrosis (dead tissue) of the genital area

(h) meatitis and meatal ulceration (affecting 20% of infants following circumcision)

(i) meatal stenosis (5% to 8% of circumcised boys, which can lead to kidney failure if untreated)

(j) penile adhesions and skin bridges

(k) phimosis requiring surgical correction (following 1% to 2% of neonatal circumcisions)

(l) retention of the Plastibell ring (if a Plastibell clamp is used, occurs in about 1-2%, resulting in painful swelling of the penis beyond the ring and possibly tissue death (necrosis) of the end of the penis)

(m) buried or concealed penis

(n) unexpected cosmetic outcomes (approximately 1% to 2% of boys undergoing a surgical revision of the circumcision to address these cosmetic concerns)

    i.   covering of the glans penis in 30% of boys

    ii.   crooked scars

    iii. rotation of the penis

    iv. scars darker or lighter than penile shaft skin

    v.   puffiness

    vi. bumps or cysts

    vii. skin tags

    viii. excessive scar tissue (keloid)

(o) partial or complete amputation of the head of the penis

(p) loss of the penis

(q) excessive penile skin loss

(r) urinary retention and obstruction (which can lead to kidney failure and bladder distention to the point of bladder rupture)

(s) lymphedema

(t) urethral fistula

(u) scrotal trauma

(v) pneumothorax

(w) unilateral leg cyanosis

(x) breath holding (approximately 1% sometimes leading to seizures)

(y) urine advancing in subcutaneous fascial planes

(z) subcutaneous granuloma (occur following 5% of circumcisions)

(aa) pyogenic granuloma

(bb) penile tourniquet syndrome (reported almost exclusively in circumcised boys in which a human hair can get wrapped around the penis, shrink and cut into or cut off the penis)

(cc) urethritis

(dd) gastric rupture

(ee) death (including increased risk of dying from sudden infant death syndrome (SIDS))

(ff) if local anesthesia is used it carries with it increased risks of

    i.   bleeding (usually small bruises at the injection sites in 1.2% to 43.5%),

    ii.   loss of blood supply to the genitals,

    iii. methemoglobinemia (associated with use of prilocaine).

14. Even when properly performed, insofar as ENTMC is painful and removes the erogenous, functional foreskin, which adolescent boys and men value, it harms all boys and men.

15. Given the facts above, it would follow that if MassHealth were to undertake an institutional review of ENTMC, it would conclude that ENTMC is not medically necessary and, as such, not a covered benefit. Given that MassHealth currently considers ENTMC a covered benefit, it appears unlikely that MassHealth has undertaken such a review.

AMERICAN ACADEMY OF PEDIATRICS

16. The 2012 circumcision policy statement of the American Academy of Pediatrics (AAP) and its supporting technical report automatically expired five years later or in 2017. The AAP did not renew its 2012 statement. There is no AAP circumcision policy statement currently in effect.

17. The 2012 circumcision policy released by the American Academy of Pediatrics has called for increased rates of reimbursement from third-party payers to those performing ENTMC.[A2] The AAP calls circumcision non-therapeutic and elective, and did not find the data from the medical literature sufficiently compelling to justify a recommendation for routine neonatal circumcision.[A3]

18. The AAP claims in its 2012 statement that "Specific benefits identified included prevention of urinary tract infections, penile cancer,
and transmission of some sexually transmitted infections, including
HIV." This is a false claim as circumcision does not prevent any of
those diseases. The AAPs real claim is that circumcision only slightly reduces the risk of boys and men acquiring those diseases, and
thus that it has a very small potential of providing a medical benefit.
Granting the AAP's claim of "potential medical benefits," it would
be necessary to expose 100 boys to the pain, risks, and harm of circumcision to prevent one urinary tract infection and between 4,000
and 7,000 boys to prevent one case of penile cancer.

19. The AAP's now-expired policy has been criticized by international
medical experts for its many factual inaccuracies and for being culturally biased reflecting the cultural normalcy of circumcision in the
United States.[A4]

20. The only potential medical benefit the AAP claims for circumcision
in childhood is a 1% reduction in the risk of acquiring a urinary tract
infection (UTI) during the first year of life. By contrast, the circumcision of infants causes meatitis and meatal ulceration in up to 20%
of cases.

21. Even granting all the AAP's claims in its 2012 circumcision policy
statement and supporting technical report, ENTMC does not qualify
as a covered Medicaid benefit. First, ENTMC is not medically necessary. Second, healthy boys are not suffering from a medical condition
requiring treatment. Third, there are not only comparable but much
more effective and more conservative ways to prevent the diseases
that the AAP discusses. For example, urinary tract infections can be
treated with oral antibiotics.[A5] Cases of penile cancer can be avoided
by vaccination, safe sexual practices, not smoking, and good penile
hygiene. Sexually transmitted infections including HIV can be prevented by monogamy, aggressive testing and treatment, pre-exposure

prophylaxis, and safe sex. Fourth, these alternative methods of disease prevention are less costly.

22. If MassHealth is relying on the AAP's 2012 circumcision policy to justify its current position, it needs to be aware that the AAP's 2012 circumcision policy statement is out of step with the rest of the world.[A6] I reviewed the AAP's 2012 30-page technical report on circumcision line by line and documented in 146 pages the ways in which I believe their report to be fatally flawed.[A7]

23. Physicians have an ethical duty to disclose conflicts of interest. The 2012 AAP circumcision policy statement failed to disclose the cultural, financial, and religious biases of the AAP and the members of its Task Force on Circumcision in favor of perpetuating the circumcision industry. Physicians who circumcise in the United States share some or all those biases.

If called as a witness, I can and will gladly testify to the facts set forth in this declaration.

I have personal knowledge of all the facts stated above and hereby swear under the pains and penalties of perjury that all of the facts in this Affidavit are true and accurate.

Further your affiant sayeth not,

Robert S. Van Howe, M.D., M.S.
Dated: July 21, 2020

A1 Citations supporting each of these claims are available upon request but take up many pages.

A2 Task Force on Circumcision. Male circumcision. *Pediatrics.* 2012;130:e756-85.

A3 Task Force on Circumcision, Cultural bias and circumcision: the AAP Task Force on Circumcision responds. *Pediatrics.* 2013;131:801-4.

A4 Cultural Bias, *supra note* 38.

A5 Hoberman A, Wald ER, Hickey RW, Baskin M, Charron M, Majd M, Kearney DH, Reynolds EA, Ruley J, Janosky JE. Oral versus initial intravenous therapy for urinary tract infections in young febrile children. *Pediatrics.* 1999;104:79-86.

A6 Svoboda JS, Van Howe RS. Out of step: fatal flaws in the latest AAP policy report on neonatal circumcision. *J Med Ethics.* 2013;39:434-41.

A7 Van Howe RS. Statement by statement analysis of the 2012 report from the American Academy of Pediatrics Task Force on Circumcision: when national organizations are guided by personal agendas II. Available at: <academia.edu/23431341>